Intermittent Fasting

The Complete Guide to Fasting for Diabetes - How to Lower Your Blood pressure and Reverse Insulin Resistance with a Few, Simple Changes in Your Diet

By

Jason Michaels

Jason Michaels

The information in the following pages is broadly considered to be a truthful and accurate account of facts and as such any inattention, use or misuse of the information in question by the reader will render any resulting actions solely under their purview. There are no scenarios in which the publisher or the original author of this work can be in any fashion deemed liable for any hardship or damages that may befall them after undertaking information described herein.

Additionally, the information in the following pages is intended only for informational purposes and should thus be thought of as universal. As befitting its nature, it is presented without assurance regarding its prolonged validity or interim quality. Trademarks that are mentioned are done without written consent and can in no way be considered an endorsement from the trademark holder.

Medical Disclaimer
This book is not intended as a substitute for the medical advice of physicians. The reader should regularly consult a physician in matters relating to his/her health and particularly with respect to any symptoms that may require diagnosis or medical attention.

Jason Michaels

Please consult your physician before starting any diet or exercise program.

Any recommendations given in this book are not a substitute for medical advice.

Contents

Introduction 9

Chapter 1: Why the Typical American Diet Is So Bad........ 11

Chapter 2: What Is Chronic Low-Grade Inflammation and

Why Does It Make You Fat?................................16

Chapter 3: Anti-Inflammatory Myths 21

Chapter 4: Top 7 Foods to Avoid 26

Chapter 5: Most Beneficial Foods and Best Anti-

inflammatory Supplements 32

Chapter 6: How to Extract the Most Nutrients from Your

Food When Cooking 38

The hidden dangers of microwaving 40

Chapter 8: Healing Foods for Leaky Gut, Arthritis, and

Other Associated Disease 50

Foods to Eat to Support Healing Leaky Gut 52
Foods to Eat to Support Arthritis 53
Types of Anti-inflammatory Foods to Eat to Help
Arthritis 54

Chapter 10: Start Feeling Better Instantly........................61

Chapter 11: Anti-inflammatory Meal Plan for 1 Week 65

Conclusion.. 70

Introduction...73

Chapter 1: What is Fasting?..75

Chapter 2: The Science Behind Intermittent Fasting........82

Chapter 3: Why Meal Timing is Irrelevant for Weight Loss

& Muscle Gain...85

Chapter 4: The Various Intermittent Fasting Structures..90

Chapter 5: Intermittent Fasting for Weight Loss 102

Chapter 6: Intermittent Fasting for Muscle Gain............105

Chapter 7: Intermittent Fasting and Exercise..................112

Chapter 8: Different Intermittent Fasting Daily Schedules

....129

Conclusion 139

Introduction..142

Chapter 1: Brief Overview of the Keto Diet 144

Fat Torch Versus Sugar Burner......................................144
Keto Diet Benefits...146
Foods to Avoid 146
Food to Embrace 147
Chapter 2: Why You Should Be Meal Prepping..............149

What is Meal Prepping?...149
Reasons Why You Should Be Meal Prepping................150

Chapter 3: How to Avoid the 10 Most Common Meal Prep

Mistakes...154

Mistake 1: Not giving yourself enough time to plan.....154
Mistake 2: Not choosing the best recipes for your
personal needs..155
Mistake 3: Being unrealistic and too ambitious...........156
Mistake 4: Not stocking the pantry 156
Mistake 5: Not searching for items that need to be used
up...158
Mistake 6: Not jotting down recipes 158
Mistake 7: Not taking inventory before shopping........159
Mistake 8: Skipping pre meal prep 159
Mistake 9: Trying new recipes each day........................160
Mistake 10: Failing to have a backup plan....................160

Chapter 4: Delicious Keto Recipes 162

Breakfast Recipes..162
Lunch Recipes 176
Mason Jar Recipes 192
Dinner Recipes..204
Dessert Recipes 221
Fat Bomb Recipes 228
Rice Alternatives 240

Emergency Keto Meals at Popular Fast Food Chains..... 242

Chapter 5: Methods to Properly Store Food....................245

Pantry Tips 245
Fridge Tips..246
Freezer Tips 247
Freezer vs. Fridge...248

Chapter 6: Meal Prep Kitchen Essentials 250

Anti-Inflammatory Diet

Make these simple, inexpensive changes to your diet and start feeling better within 24 hours!

By

Jason Michaels

Introduction

Congratulations on downloading Anti-Inflammatory Diet:
Make these simple, inexpensive changes to your diet and
start feeling better within 24 hours! and thank you for
doing so.

The following chapters will discuss **how** the anti-
inflammatory diet isn't a diet in the traditional meaning of
the term, because its intended purpose isn't weight loss,
though people do often lose weight when following it. It's
also not a diet you follow for a limited time until you reach
your goal and then quit. Rather it's a true lifestyle change
focused on anti-inflammatory principles with the purpose
of providing stable energy, and adequate vitamins,
essential fatty acids, minerals, fiber, and defensive anti-
inflammatory phytonutrients to reach and maintain better
health.

This book is written to help people understand aspects of
inflammation and how the typical American diet
contributes to it. It looks at the effects of the resulting
chronic inflammation on health and how chronic low-
grade inflammation can even contribute to weight gain and
other health issues. Once equipped with this
understanding, you'll learn what you can do about it with a

goal to consume less processed and fast foods and more fresh whole foods including plenty of fruits and vegetables. The entire focus of the anti-inflammatory diet is health and healing your body's ailments.

This book also navigates through and beyond misinformation and myths surrounding the diet and lays the groundwork for your new lifestyle. It explains the variety of foods to eat for healing, what foods to avoid, and the best ways to cook meals to get the most benefit. In the end, you'll be equipped with the information you need to get started and to noticeably feel better including a one-week meal plan to get you on track.

There are plenty of books on this subject on the market, thanks again for choosing this one! Every effort was made to ensure it is full of as much useful information as possible, please enjoy!

Thanks,
Jason

Chapter 1: Why the Typical American Diet Is So Bad

Statistics available through the U.S. Department of Health & Human Services (HSS) shine a light on how bad the typical American diet is for us. For starters, "it exceeds the recommended intake levels or limits in four categories: calories from solid fats and added sugars; refined grains; sodium; and saturated fat." All this directly affects your health. In fact, the HSS says that "if Americans reduced the sodium they eat by 1,200 mg per day" going forward "it would save up to $20 billion a year in medical costs." We now get an astonishing 63% of our calories from refined or process foods. And while we eat too much of those foods, on the other end of the spectrum, Americans don't consume the recommended amounts of fruits, vegetables, whole-grains, and healthy oils. In fact, only 12% of our calories coming from plant-based foods. When you look at that statistic even closer, it's even worse because half of that already-low percentage comes from French fries. That means the real number of healthy plant-based foods is reduced to 6%, a figure that can only be described as horrifyingly low.

According to the HSS, calories containing no nutrients coming from solid fats and added sugars in the typical American diet "contribute to 40% of the total daily calories for 2 – 18-year-olds and half of these empty calories come from six sources: soda, fruit drinks, dairy desserts, grain desserts, pizza, and whole milk." Forty percent of daily calories! This means almost half of their daily calories contain little or no real nutrients because they are derived from these solid fats and added sugars. And what about the rest of us? Out of a 2775 daily calorie diet, the USDA estimated that in 2010 nearly 1,000 calories a day come from added fats and sweeteners, while only 424 calories came from dairy, fruits, and vegetables.

To better understand what we are talking about, it helps to understand that solid fats are fats that solidify at room temperature. This includes fats like butter, shortening, and fats that cook off of beef, pork, and other meats. Solid fats can be added when foods are processed by manufacturers or when they are prepared for consumption in restaurants or home. In the same way, added sugars include various types of sugars and syrups which are added when foods or beverages are processed or prepared.

In the last 65 years, the amount of sugar we consume has radically gone up, and along with that, the origin of where we get the sugar has also drastically changed. In the 1950s, Americans mostly ate sugar derived from sugarcane and sugar beets, but the year 2000, the USDA reports that each individual in America took in 150 pounds of sugar a year with more than half of that coming from corn in the form of high fructose corn syrup. And no, just because it comes from the plant corn does not make it a sweetener that's good for your health.

Over the last century, our palates have transformed along with the ingredients in our food. Just look at the ingredients list on the foods you buy. Ingredients are listed in the order of prevalence, with ingredients added in the greatest amount listed first, followed in descending order by those in smaller amounts. Sugar in one of its forms is often listed in the first three, because today with the typical American diet everything we eat needs to be really sweet, including foods we don't typically consider sweet such as bread. While sugar is needed to get the yeast to activate and ferment, if you check the label on that multi-grain bread, each slice provides 2.6 grams of sugar from honey and refined sugar.

What's more is, as you read the product label, sugar can be listed by numerous names. These names include anhydrous dextrose, cane juice, corn sweetener, corn syrup, dextrose, fructose, high-fructose corn syrup, corn syrup solids, invert sugar, malt syrup, maltose, lactose, sucrose and white sugar. Unfortunately, food manufacturers aren't required to separate added sugar from naturally occurring sugar but are only required to divulge total over-all sugars per serving.

With the consumption of all these empty calories, today more than 1 in 3 adults suffer from pre-diabetes. This condition happens as the result of higher than "normal" blood sugar levels which aren't at levels bad enough to be identified as type 2 diabetes. Plus, 30 million Americans are inflicted with diabetes but 1 out of 4 aren't even conscious of it.

The bottom line is that Americans aren't taking in enough vital nutrients, fiber, and natural fats needed to attain the best health. This is really sad when you think about how prosperous this great country is and yet we experience higher rates of disease than other developed nations.

What's the cumulative effect of the typical American diet over time? In a nutshell, the standard American diet can lead to chronic inflammation which leads to progressive tissue damage and inflammatory diseases like rheumatoid arthritis and leaky gut. Others ailments include what is known as "unexplained symptoms". These include things like headaches, brain fog, bleeding gums, allergies, fatigue, mood swings, and skin rashes. In other words, random aches and pains that you can't identify the cause of. In the following chapters, we will take a closer look at chronic low-grade inflammation and what it does to the body. What does this all mean for you? Well simply put, many of your health problems could be caused by nothing more than the food you put into your body on a daily basis. Along with things like causing joint pain, it could well be the reason you're struggling with your weight!

Chapter 2: What Is Chronic Low-Grade Inflammation and Why Does It Make You Fat?

Chronic pain is a growing problem in America. People struggle to get through the day as they battle conditions like arthritis, fibromyalgia, back pain, and more. Many seek relief through strong prescription medication and while this may offer relief, it may also result in unwanted side effects. For those who would rather find another answer, a more natural answer, it's key to understand the connection linking inflammation and pain and the food we put in our mouth. Diets full of things like gluten, trans-fats, pasteurized dairy, corn (including corn sweeteners), and soy are at the source of the pain and inflammation – the same inflammation causing other medical conditions including overweight and obesity.

If you're battling your weight, even though you've cut calories, are exercising regularly and have stopped eating after 8 p.m., have you wondered why you're still carrying all that extra weight around your middle? It just might be that as hard as you are fighting to lose that excess weight, your body is fighting to keep it. Why? Chronic, low-grade inflammation caused by what you are eating.

To understand what one has to do with the other, first, we have to understand chronic inflammation. It is your body's bewildered and detrimental immune response to your environment. Which including poor diet, stress, allergens, and toxic substances. Research shows that what we eat is a significant contributor to chronic inflammation and our gut health. Other factors that contribute to chronic inflammation include a sedentary lifestyle and chronic stress, and living with hidden infections (including things like gum disease).

All these factors trigger this unseen inflammation running deep within our cells and tissues. Think of it like a smoldering fire and when we eat the wrong foods, all we're doing is feeding that fire. And when cytokines that respond to this unseen inflammation fill the bloodstream, it can lead to systemic inflammation, which in turn can lead to cardiovascular diseases. Cholesterol deposits cling to the lining of inflamed blood vessels and grow with a fatty plaque which can lead to blockages and blood clots which in turn can lead to a heart attack.

In this book, we will focus on the dietary link to inflammation, because over time, the continual inflammatory response to our diet is what can lead to

Jason Michaels

weight gain and digestive issues. HHS reports that it is
projected that "by 2030, half of all adults (115 million
adults) in the United States will be obese." While normal
inflammation is a good thing that works to protect and heal
your body, chronic or systemic inflammation happens
when your immune system gets out of balance and instead
of healing, it contributes to disease and weight gain. The
sugar we eat contributes to this shift in balance but it isn't
the only culprit. Eating the wrong oils and fats including
processed seed- and vegetable oils like soybean and corn
oil, and hidden food allergens also contribute to the
problem.

The influence of food allergens is the culprit directly
related to weight gain. We're not talking about life-
threatening food allergies some people have to specific
foods like peanuts or shellfish, but is a different kind of
reaction called a delayed allergy (IgG delated
hypersensitivity reaction). This kind of deferred response
may result in symptoms within a few hours or can be
delayed for a few days after eating. This is a much more
common allergy and leads millions of people to suffer
because it plays a big part in numerous chronic ailments as
well as problems with weight. In fact, it's a major
contributor to obesity.

So, if you are on the older end of middle age or younger and struggling with your weight even though you think you're doing all the right things, then chronic inflammation could be the cause and an anti-inflammation diet the answer. Eating anti-inflammatory foods eliminates foods containing hidden food allergens and sensitivities, and can help you lose that stubborn weight effectively and permanently as long as you continue to eat the right foods.

Chronic inflammation wears down your immune system over time because it is on-going. As your body continually responds to this inflammation, it eventually leads to chronic diseases and other health issues including:

- Allergies which contribute to sinus and nasal congestion, weight gain, fluid retention, fatigue, joint pains, acne, eczema, brain fog, irritable bowel syndrome (IBS), mood issues, headaches
- Arthritis
- Asthma
- Autoimmune diseases
- Cancer
- Osteoporosis
- Premature aging

Jason Michaels

Regrettably, most often these chronic health challenges are treated with drugs and/or surgery, which may or may not offer temporary relief from symptoms, but these solutions don't actually address the root of the problem. But if you shop for the right doctor, today you can find an integrative MD who is willing to not only identify health issues but to address them by taking into consideration your lifestyle for ways to eliminate behaviors that lead to chronic inflammation. You can even ask them to run a CRP (C-reactive Protein test) to test your blood for a C-reactive protein which is a blood test marker for inflammation. It forms in the liver and is classified as an "acute phase reactant," which means levels grow higher in as a result of inflammation.

Chapter 3: Anti-Inflammatory Myths

While you can find plenty of information about eating to reduce inflammation, you'll also find plenty of myths and misinformation surrounding the anti-inflammatory diet, too. These myths include warning about foods to avoid as well as foods to eat, along with general all-encompassing statements like everything on the diet tastes terrible, or it's too expensive, so it's important to be informed so you don't sabotage your efforts toward better health before you really get started.

The myths listed in this chapter are deemed so because there's no scientific evidence to support them.

Myth #1: Citrus Fruits Bring About Inflammation

The need to ban citrus fruits because they cause inflammation is one of those unsubstantiated myths circulating on several online forums. The chatter condemns this fruit with little to no scientific evidence to back up claims. In truth, citrus is loaded with vitamin C and proven to reduce the progression of Osteoarthritis. Vitamin C is a beneficial antioxidant and citrus is also known to play an important part in the formation of cartilage.

Myth #2: A Raw Food Diet Alleviates Inflammation

While eating more fruits and vegetables is a good direction to go, eating an all-raw diet isn't necessarily the best solution to fight inflammation. A sudden change in diet like going all raw can actually help promote inflammation instead of relieving it, and the bacteria in your gut may have trouble processing foods so far out of your normal range of choices.

Myth 3: Gin-soaked Raisins Ease Symptoms

This myth is an old wives' tale that finds its origins in the hype surrounding the healing properties of juniper berries which are used to make gin combined with the belief that the sulfur in raisins eases joint pain. And while there may be an inkling of truth in this, it is an unrealistic claim because the amounts typically eaten are so small they make no real impact on your inflammation affecting joints.

Myth #4: Eating a Diet High in Fish Is the Same as Taking AlphaFlex or Fish Oil Supplements

Sorry to say, diet alone can't take the place of AlphaFlex® or other anti-inflammatory supplements. Although the

Omega-3's found in fish have anti-inflammatory properties, you would have to eat a large quantity of fish to try to match the anti-inflammatory power of a supplement but you couldn't do it. Plus, fish can also be high in mercury, and excessive consumption could lead to the potential of mercury poisoning.

Myth 5: Eating a low-acid diet helps avoid arthritis flare-ups

The thinking behind this myth says to avoid foods high in acid, like citrus fruits and tomatoes to minimize pain and flare-ups. The problem with this is that as you eat and drink gets balanced once it enters your stomach. The digestive system adjusts foods whether acidic and alkaline and neutralizes and supposed benefit or detriment based on those qualifiers. Plus, citrus fruits are high in vitamin C which works as an anti-inflammatory.

Myth 6: Making Healthier Choices Is Cost Prohibitive

And one more myth related to following the anti-inflammatory diet is that healthier choices are cost prohibitive. It is true that processed foods filled with added sugars and higher fat content do cost less monetarily than nutrient-dense whole fruits, vegetables, lean meats. In fact,

Jason Michaels

fresh vegetable and fruit prices rose almost 120% from
1985 – 2000. With those kinds of statistics, it does seem
like making healthier choices is just too expensive for some
of us. But that's really not the case.

Findings in a recent meta-analysis by researchers at Brown
University and the Harvard School of Public Health shine a
light on just how much more expensive it really is to buy
healthier food options. They crunched numbers from 27
previous studies and what did they find? The cost for an
adult to eat healthy comes to $1.48 a day more than eating
a poor-quality diet. That calculates out to $550 more per
person a year. Isn't that worth it for better health?

There are a few ways that can help you save more when
eating a healthy anti-inflammatory diet. One of the big
ones is to eat out less and to cook for yourself more. For
instance, people spend an average of $11 per meal eating
lunch out, but only $6.30 on average when they prepare
their own lunch, plus when you make your own food you
have the added benefit of knowing exactly what is in it.
Also, as you increase the amount of fruits and vegetables in
your diet, you'll find if you buy them in season you'll get
the best value.

One last myth worth mentioning, even though it doesn't have anything to do with food and nutrition, is that all anti-inflammatory medications have minimal side effects. Sadly, the opposite is true. Even anti-inflammatory over-the-counter drugs like ibuprofen, naproxen, Celebrex and other non-steroidal drugs can result in a number of side effects, plus these drugs really need to be taken in prescription doses to curb inflammation. These possible side effects include ulcers that may possibly become life-threatening, abdominal pain, diarrhea, dry mouth, kidney failure, swelling, and dizziness. On the flip side, fish oil is a natural supplement that fights inflammation without any known adverse side effects. When searching for a fish oil, you should choose one that has the optimal EPA/DHA ratio. Ideally you want a supplement with 180mg EPA and 120mg DHA per serving.

Jason Michaels

Chapter 4: Top 7 Foods to Avoid

When eating to reduce inflammation, it is best to avoid most packaged foods because they contain inflammation-triggering preservatives, colorings, and artificial flavorings to increase their shelf life. If it is packaged in a box or bag, chances are that it's not good for your health. Eating too many inflammatory foods can lead to chronic low-grade inflammation which in turn can cause serious health issues including cancer, heart disease, diabetes, and allergies. With that said, this chapter looks at seven specific inflammatory foods to avoid.

1. Gluten and Wheat

As we've already discussed, inflammation is the natural response of your immune system. When we get a splinter, inflammation makes the surrounding area red and tender. With this picture in mind, let's look at why you should avoid gluten.

Proteins found in wheat are gut irritants, and the term "gluten" is a general name for these proteins. Now, picture tiny splinters raking into the lining of your gut and resulting in inflammation. When it comes to gluten, the most well-known gluten-related inflammation is celiac disease or non-celiac gluten sensitivity, but wheat can also be a problem for people who aren't specifically sensitive to gluten because of amylase trypsin inhibitors (ATIs) found in wheat. These ATIs can bring about an inflammatory immune response in the GI tract which contributes to another problem called intestinal permeability, or leaky gut, which we will cover more in chapter 8. This condition lets undigested food particles, bacteria, and toxic waste products "leak" through the intestines into your bloodstream.

2. Refined Carbohydrates

Carbohydrates are commonly referred to as "good" and "bad." Complex carbs are good because they are filled with beneficial fiber. When it comes to inflammation, refined carbohydrates fall into the bad category because in the refining process most of their fiber is removed. With the fiber removed, refined carbs raise blood sugar levels and raise the occurrence of inflammatory changes. This influence can lead to disease. For instance, when looking at our modern diet, research has shown refined carbs can encourage the development of inflammatory bacteria in the gut which can raise the probability of obesity and IBS.

3. Milk Lactose

Jason Michaels

Milk lactose is a sugar found in milk which causes digestive issues for many people because their bodies don't produce the lactase enzyme required to digest it. Other people who do produce this enzyme may still react poorly to drinking milk because of the proteins casein and whey. Casein actually has a molecular structure very similar to gluten, and half the people who can't tolerate gluten don't tolerate casein well either. As a result, dairy is one of the most inflammatory foods in today's diet, second only to gluten. Adverse digestive symptoms resulting from this inflammation may manifest in bloating, constipation, diarrhea, and gas. Other non-digestive symptoms include acne and a compelling demonstration of autistic behaviors. So lactose is only half the issue when it comes to milk and milk products, the others are the casein and whey proteins.

A study also showed that women in China have a far lower rate of breast cancer than women in the West. The only noticeable difference between the two diets is lower milk intake. A Harvard professor has also discovered links between ovarian cancer and dairy consumption.

4. Sugar

It's no secret that eating too many added sugars and refined carbohydrates can lead to overweight and obesity, but the consequences of eating excesses are also linked to increased gut permeability, raised inflammatory markers, and high LDL cholesterol. The thing all these factors have in common is that they can trigger low-grade chronic inflammation. Excess body fat, especially belly fat, results in continuous, chronic levels of inflammation which can modify how insulin works. Insulin, as a regulatory hormone, plays a big part in carrying the glucose in your bloodstream into your cells for energy, but when blood glucose levels are chronically high, the production and regulation of insulin is changed resulting in insulin resistance. The resulting overabundance of blood glucose can lead to an accumulation of advanced glycation end products (AGEs). When too many AGEs bind with our cells and integral proteins, it can lead to oxidative stress and inflammation. It can change their structure, inhibit their regular function and eventually result in a buildup of arterial plaque and decreased kidney function, among other things.

5. Meat

Grain fed beef has been touted as tasting better, but cows are naturally grazers that eat grass. When fed grain they grow fat quickly before they are sold by the pound for profit. Cattle, pigs, and chickens are not naturally grain eaters. But in life on the feed-lot not only are they fed things like corn and soy, they are also given antibiotics to make sure they don't get sick. This translates to meats on our dinner table that are not only higher in inflammatory saturated fats but also contain higher levels of inflammatory omega-6s from their unnatural diet. To compound the problem, when we grill our meat at high temperatures, it results in inflammatory carcinogens! So if you plan to eat meat, choose grass-fed varieties.

.

6. Saturated Fats

When you think saturated fats, many people think of red meat, but aside from fatty cuts of beef, saturated fat is also found in pork and lamb, the skin of chicken, as well as processed meats. It's also found in dairy products like butter, cream (including whipped cream), cheese, and regular-fat milk. Studies have linked the consumption of saturated fats with causing the kind of body fat that stores energy rather than burns it. As these fat cells grow bigger they release pro-inflammatory drivers that promote systemic inflammation.

7. Alcohol

Drinking alcohol puts a burden on the liver, and when consumed in excess, it weakens liver function. This disrupts other multi-organ interactions resulting in inflammation. If you choose to drink alcohol, do so in moderation, but it is best eliminated if you're fighting inflammation.

Chapter 5: Most Beneficial Foods and Best Anti-inflammatory Supplements

Many conditions can be traced back to inflammation. Joint pain, autoimmune disorders, irritable bowel syndrome (IBS), mood imbalances, acne, and eczema are just a few conditions that can be linked back to inflammation. Once the origin of inflammation is identified, an anti-inflammatory diet can help ease symptoms and certain foods and supplements can help lessen the inflammation in your body. In this chapter, we'll list some of the best minerals and beneficial antioxidants found in foods and supplements to add to your arsenal to fight inflammation. This list is arranged in alphabetical order to make it easier to use as a reference tool.

Blueberries

Blueberries make the list as an antioxidant superfood. This dark, delicious fruit may be small, but it's crammed with antioxidants and phytoflavinoids. These tiny berries are high in potassium and vitamin C and work as an anti-inflammatory to aid in lowering the risk of heart disease and cancer. Strawberries, raspberries, and blackberries also contain anthocyanins which provide anti-inflammatory effects.

Avocado

Avocados are packed with potassium, magnesium, and fiber. This savory fruit is another superfood rich in antioxidants and anti-inflammatory properties. They provide a great source of healthy unsaturated fat and are packed with potassium, magnesium, and fiber.

Coenzyme Q10

Coenzyme Q10, also known as CoQ10, is another antioxidant that shown to offer anti-inflammatory properties. It is found naturally in avocados, olive oil, parsley, peanuts, beef liver, salmon, sardines, mackerel, spinach, and walnuts.

Ginger

Ginger is comparative to in that contains powerful anti-inflammatory compounds known as gingerols. Ginger root is found in the produce section at your grocery store and is available as a potent antioxidant supplement that helps prevent the oxidation of a damaging free radical called peroxynitrite. Ginger adds flavor to your favorite stir-fry, can be made into ginger tea, or can be taken as a supplement.

Glutathione

Glutathione is another antioxidant that fights free-radicals with anti-inflammatory properties. This is available as a supplement and is also available naturally in plant foods including apples, asparagus, avocados, garlic, grapefruit, spinach, tomatoes, and milk thistle.

Magnesium

Magnesium is a mineral supplement that can help reduce inflammation for those with low magnesium which is linked to stress. Statistics suggest an estimated 70% of Americans are deficient in this mineral which is surprising since it is readily available in a number of foods including dark leafy greens, almonds, avocado, and many legumes.

Salmon

Salmon is rich in anti-inflammatory omega-3s. It is better to eat wild caught than farmed. It is best to try to include oily fish in your diet two times a week, and if you're not a fan of fish, then try a high-quality fish oil supplement.

Turmeric/Curcumin

Turmeric is the yellow spice that gives curry its color, and curcumin is the active ingredient in turmeric and can be purchased as a supplement. The two words are often used interchangeably, but curcumin is the key ingredient which offers powerful anti-inflammatory effects. It's a strong antioxidant and as a powdered spice, turmeric can be added to soups and curries, and curcumin can be taken in supplement form.

Vitamin B

People with low levels of vitamin B6 have a tendency to have high levels of C-reactive protein which, as was mentioned in chapter 2, is a measure of inflammation in the body. B vitamins, including B6, can be found in vegetables like broccoli, bell peppers, cauliflower, kale, and mushrooms. It is also available in meats including chicken, cod, turkey, and tuna.

Folate (B-9 in natural form) and folic acid (a synthetic form of B-9) is another B vitamin linked to the reduction of inflammation. A brief Italian study submits that even daily, short-term low dosages of folic acid supplements can lessen inflammation in overweight people. Folate is found in foods like asparagus, black-eyed peas, dark leafy greens, and lima beans.

Vitamin D

Estimates suggest two-thirds of the people living in the U.S. are deficient in vitamin D. It's another vitamin that helps reduce inflammation, and getting insufficient amounts is linked to a range of inflammatory conditions. This vitamin is unique in that we get it naturally when we spend time in the sunshine with the important spectrum is ultraviolet B (UVB). It is also available as a supplement and is available in foods like egg yolks, fish and organ meats, as well as foods that are supplemented with it. When choosing a Vitamin D supplement, look for Vitamin D3, which is the most bioavailable form of the vitamin. The ideal amount for supplementation is 5000IU per day, and many of this pills cost less than $7 for a 3 month supply.

Vitamin E

Another potent antioxidant, this vitamin can aid in lessening inflammation. It is available as a quality supplement or can be found naturally in nuts and seeds, and vegetables like avocado and spinach.

Vitamin K

There are two kinds of vitamin K: K1 and K2. K1 is found in leafy greens, cabbage, and cauliflower. K2 is available in eggs and liver. This vitamin helps reduce inflammatory markers and may help to fight osteoporosis and heart disease.

Chapter 6: How to Extract the Most Nutrients from Your Food When Cooking

For decades, raw foodists have warned that cooking not only kills vitamins and minerals in food but also denatures the enzymes that help us digest the foods we eat. We've heard this for so long, many of us had embraced it as fact, but the truth is raw vegetables aren't always healthier, and in some cases, cooking is actually important if we want to get the most nutritional benefit from the foods we eat. Cooking can help us digest food without spending volumes of energy and makes foods like cellulose fiber and raw meat softer for and easier for our digestive systems to handle.

It turns out that vegetables like asparagus, cabbage, carrots, peppers, mushrooms, spinach, and numerous others, actually supply our bodies with more antioxidants like carotenoids and ferulic acid when boiled or steamed as opposed to raw. A January 2008 report in the Journal of Agriculture and Food Chemistry reported that when cooking vegetables "boiling and steaming preserved antioxidants better than frying." This was mainly the case with carotenoid present in broccoli, carrots, and zucchini.

And before you shrug it off and say, "Any cooking method is better than frying," it's important to note that researchers actually examined the effect of several cooking methods on compounds such as carotenoids, polyphenols, and ascorbic acid and determined boiling to be the best way to extract these nutrients for consumption.

In the same year, a study published in The British Journal of Nutrition backed up this cooking benefit claim. This study consisted of a group of 198 participants and found those who adhered to an inflexible raw food diet showed normal quantities of vitamin A and comparatively elevated levels of beta-carotene. However, they had low levels of the antioxidant lycopene, a carotenoid with anti-inflammatory properties. Remember, these are findings for eating raw. In contrast, another study published in the Journal of Agriculture and Food Chemistry found that cooking essentially raises the quantity of lycopene in tomatoes. "The level of one type of lycopene, cis-lycopene, rose 35% after being cooked for 30 minutes at 190.4 degrees Fahrenheit." The conclusions drawn suggest that heat causes the thick cell walls of the plant to break down which aids in the body's absorption of nutrients which were bound to those cell walls.

So now that we know some nutrition is enhanced by cooking but not everything is best cooked, it leaves us with the question: "What should I cook and what should I eat raw on the anti-inflammatory diet?" The fact is that each food is a little different. The raw foodist mentality holds that many foods high in antioxidants are sensitive to cooking because phytonutrients don't hold up well to high temperatures and when it reaches the "heat labile point" it results in a change that causes foods to lose enzymes beneficial to us. But this is only half the story. The truth is that whether you should eat a vegetable cooked or raw for the most nutritional benefit depends on the vegetable and the way you cook it.

The hidden dangers of microwaving

Before we go any further, let's be clear – deep frying offers no benefit, and microwaving your food can actually bring about an inflammatory response. This is because microwaving brings about a change in the chemical structure of your food. In fact, it so completely alters the protein structure of food that the body doesn't even recognize it as a food, but instead looks at as a foreign toxin which warrants an inflammatory response.

Microwaving food is also harmful to nutritive benefit and leads to a loss of up to 90% of the nutritional value. It converts tasty, organic vegetables into nutritionally "dead" food that can bring about disease because microwaving changes plant alkaloids into carcinogens. Take garlic for example. It's a powerful healing food when eaten raw and is of great benefit to digestive health, cellular immunity, heart health and more, but when microwaved for just 60 seconds the active component, allinase, become inactive. So the very component known to help protect against cancer is no longer any benefit at all.

The same kinds of changes occur when microwaving grains and milk, too. In these cases, the amino acids are converted into carcinogenic substances. When it comes to prepared meats microwaving again results in the development of cancer-causing agents. And if you use the microwave to thaw frozen fruits, it causes the sugar molecule to break down into carcinogenic substances.

An additional concern deals with carcinogenic toxins which can leach out of plastic containers, lids, or wraps used when microwaving. One of the nastiest contaminants is BPA which can cause chaos with our natural hormone levels. Often, BPAs can overstimulate the manufacture of oestrogen which can lead to oestrogenic cancers. So the next time you think about popping your food into the microwave, remember that microwaving results in molecular damage which not only kills nutritional benefits, but in its wake, leaves carcinogenic substances. So while it can seem convenient to rapidly heat your food, microwaving is not worth the nutritional loss or risk to your health.

Cooking with light heat or steam is the best as it breaks down food making it release easier-to-absorb nutrients. In some cases, as we've seen, it can even increase the nutrient content available. Another benefit related to cooking is that it can also transform chemicals from being potentially harmful to harmless. But, it depends on the vegetable and the method of cooking.

With all this in mind, the following list of vegetables is the ones better eaten cooked.

Asparagus:

The best way to cook asparagus is to steam or blanch it or bake it in a casserole. The process breaks down the fibrous spears making them easier to digest and allowing easier absorption of nutrients including vitamins A, B, C, E, and K.

Broccoli:

Finding the best way to cook broccoli is a little trickier. Those who have hypothyroidism, shouldn't eat your broccoli raw because it contains a thyroid-disrupting element. Steaming lets you preserve the nutrients while leaching out some of this element. Also, to retain a healthy amount of beneficial elements of broccoli, it helps to chop it before steaming. Avoid microwaving or boiling.

Carrots:

Carrots are best cooked by roasting or steaming. As the study mentioned earlier revealed, cooking your carrots can significantly raise the bioavailability of beta-carotene which is converted to vitamin A in our bodies. When you eat carrots raw, it's not absorbed as well.

Red Peppers:

When preparing red peppers roasting is the most advantageous. These vegetables are a remarkable source of carotenoids. And, like carrots, cooking can enhance the bioavailability of these carotenoids. However, don't

Jason Michaels

overcook because it can destroy heat-sensitive antioxidants.

Spinach:

Dark green spinach leaves make a popular salad choice, but it turns out this is another vegetable that is better eaten cooked. Nutritionally, it's best to steam it. Because it wilts when steamed, one cup steamed holds more actual spinach as well as nutrients than one cup raw. But there's another cooking benefit related to the oxalic acid found in spinach. Oxalic acid hampers the absorption of certain minerals including calcium and iron and can even develop kidney stones. But cooking spinach reduces oxalic acid by 5—53%, and if you boil it, the percentage lost rises to 30—37%. However, steaming is better unless you are prone to kidney stones because boiling leaches folate from spinach leaves.

Tomatoes:

Tomatoes are a rich source of lycopene which offers both anti-inflammatory and antioxidant properties and it, too, becomes more bioavailable after cooking. Just cook them with a little olive oil, or reduce tomatoes down to a sauce, tomato puree, or ketchup to notably increase the absorption of lycopene.

Chapter 7: Foods You Wouldn't Have Thought Were Good for You

It isn't uncommon when starting a diet to think, you'll have to give up everything you like, but with the anti-inflammatory diet, you may be pleasantly surprised to find there are delicious anti-inflammatory food and drinks options on the menu that you wouldn't have thought good for you.

Dark Chocolate

Let's start with chocolate. It not only makes for a special treat, it is actually good for you! When choosing chocolate with anti-inflammatory benefits look for chocolate that contains at least 70% cocoa (at the minimum). Along with being loaded with antioxidants that reduce inflammation, it may also lead to healthier aging because the flavonoids found in dark chocolate modify the production of a pro-inflammatory cytokine. Research suggests eating dark chocolate regularly or even occasionally can bring about beneficial results on blood pressure, oxidative stress, vascular damage, and insulin resistance.

Coffee

Jason Michaels

More than half of people in the United States drink coffee every day, but should we? Turns out coffee is actually the chief source of antioxidants in American diets. So it's okay to look forward to that cup of coffee in the morning for more than one reason whether it's decaf or regular because it contains polyphenols and other anti-inflammatory compounds. Numerous studies back this up, but one published in 2015 discovered that "over 30 years, nonsmokers who drank 3 to 5 cups of coffee a day were 15 percent less likely to die of any cause compared to people who didn't drink coffee." The coffee drinkers showed lower rates of death from heart disease, stroke, and neural conditions.

However, there is a downside to drinking coffee for some people as it causes some to experience insomnia, anxiety, irregular heartbeat and other negative side effects like irritation of the digestive system. If you experience any downside to drinking coffee, then it is best to avoid it. Try tea instead.

Tea
Green tea is another good-for-you beverage option. Of the many green teas available, Matcha tea is the most nutrient-rich. It offers up to 17 times more antioxidants than found in wild blueberries, and seven times more than what is in

dark chocolate. What may surprise you, though, is that green, white or black tea all enjoy potent anti-inflammatory benefits. So if you're not a fan of green tea, you can drink the tea of your choice and still get the potent anti-inflammatory benefits of catechin polyphenols.

Garlic and Onions

Garlic and onions bring plenty of flavor to the anti-inflammatory food palate. Garlic has a long history as a staple folk treatment for colds and other illness. It provides sulfur compounds that encourage the immune system to battle disease. Garlic has been shown to work in the same way as over the counter nonsteroidal anti-inflammatory pain drugs like ibuprofen, by reducing pathways that lead to inflammation.

Onions provide comparable anti-inflammatory compounds, one of which is the phytonutrient quercetin, which breaks down to create free radical-fighting sulfenic acid. Crushing and chopping garlic and onion releases the enzyme alliinase, which helps form a nutrient called allicin. When consumed, allicin helps form other compounds that may protect us against disease.

Fermented Foods

Jason Michaels

If you're new to fermented foods they open a whole new experience in taste. Kombucha is a fermented lightly sweetened effervescent drink that's fermented. It's made with black or green tea and boasts a host of health benefits. You can buy kombucha in the cooler section of many stores, or if you're a DIY person, you can buy a kit or active Kombucha Scoby and you're your own. Along with kombucha, fermented dishes or products to try include kefir, miso, and sauerkraut. These cultured foods provide healthy bacteria which will optimize your gut health and support a healthy immune system, which in turn helps to reduce inflammation in the body.

In some ways, learning to follow an anti-inflammatory diet is a journey as you unlearn past behaviors and reinvent your tastes as to what is really good. Keep nuts like nuts like almonds and walnuts on hand for a go-to snack along with a selection of fruits like strawberries, blueberries, cherries, pineapple, and oranges.

Strawberries in particular are great if you're searching for a flat stomach. These delicious berries are packed with polyphenols which a study by the Texas Women's University found decreased the formation of fat cells in the stomach by up to 73%.

Yes, making changes to avoid inflammation does take some work and a change in thinking, and in some cases a change in the preferences of your taste buds, but when you realize you can enjoy foods you really like that actually heal your body and improve your health and even your mood and can save you money on drugs, you'll embrace the change.

Chapter 8: Healing Foods for Leaky Gut, Arthritis, and Other Associated Disease

We've talked about how the anti-inflammatory diet is a healing diet and, in this chapter, we will take a closer look at what that really means for people with leaky gut and arthritis. For many of us, looking at inflammation as a root cause is a new concept, because traditionally modern medicine treats it as a symptom. For instance, we know arthritis is inflammation of the joints. The common answer is to take medication to reduce inflammation, but that's only treating the symptom and isn't really addressing the real problem – what's causing the inflammation. When health professionals discuss an anti-inflammatory diet, this type of low-grade, chronic inflammation is what they normally expect to help.

Before we take a closer look at arthritis and what anti-inflammatory foods to eat to specifically to help combat that condition, we will discuss another condition that can leave you feeling depressed, fatigued, anxious, struggling with weight problems or digestive symptoms. We're talking about leaky gut syndrome which is also identified as increased intestinal permeability. It's a dangerous health condition in which your digestive tract gets damaged and permits bad bacteria, proteins like gluten, and undigested bits of food to pass into your bloodstream. Some of the early symptoms of leaky gut can include skin conditions like acne and eczema, food allergies, and digestive issues including bloating, gas and irritable bowel syndrome (IBS). Over time leaky gut causes systemic inflammation and an immune reaction. It's been associated with chronic diseases and conditions including asthma, autism, chronic fatigue syndrome, depression, diabetes, heart failure, IBS, infertility, kidney disease, lupus, multiple sclerosis, narcolepsy, psoriasis, rheumatoid arthritis, and more.

Most people don't begin to understand the role our intestines play in our overall health. The small intestine absorbs the majority of the vitamins and minerals from the foods we eat. For this absorption to take place, the small intestine is equipped with tiny pores that allow nutrients to be transferred into the bloodstream. The bloodstream works as a conduit that carries and deposits these nutrients around the body. Because the intestine has these tiny pores, the wall of the intestine is referred to as semi-permeable because it permits specific things like nutrients and other beneficial molecules to enter the bloodstream while blocking things like toxins and undigested food particles.

An unhealthy small intestine suffering from leak gut no longer works properly because the pores widen and allow harmful things to pass into your bloodstream and to be transported throughout the body. Often the body starts to recognize certain foods as toxic which results in an immune reaction every time you eat that food. If the problem goes on unchecked, leaky gut can advance to an autoimmune disease. To repair this increased intestinal permeability specific diet changes must be made.

Foods to Eat to Support Healing Leaky Gut

Foods that help leaky gut are easy to digest and can aid in healing the lining of the intestines:

Bone broth: Delivers important amino acids and minerals that can aid in healing heal leaky gut and improve mineral deficits. Best if made from scratch.
Probiotic-rich foods: Raw cultured dairy products like yogurt, kefir, and amasai can help heal the gut by wiping out bad bacteria.

Healthy fats: Consume healthy fats found in foods like avocados, egg yolks, coconut oil, salmon, and ghee in moderation. These fats promote healing and are easy on the gut.

Fermented vegetables: Foods like sauerkraut, kimchi, coconut kefir, or kvass contain probiotics vital in mending leaky gut by balancing the pH in the stomach and small intestines.

Steamed vegetables: Steamed non-starchy vegetables are easy to digest and a crucial part of the leaky gut diet. Fruit: Fruit should be eaten in moderation; 1-2 servings each day. Best to eat it in the morning.

Foods to Eat to Support Arthritis

When the body is inflamed, C-reactive protein levels (CRP) rise, so if present it's a clear indicator of inflammation. Doctors can order a test checking for CRPs. According to studies published in Molecular Nutrition & Food Research and in the Journal of Nutrition, whole grains such as brown rice, bulgur, quinoa, and others have been linked with reduced CRP levels. Another study in the Journal of Nutrition discovered that people who ate smaller amounts of whole grains essentially experienced higher inflammation markers. According to the Arthritis

Jason Michaels

Foundation, the fiber available in whole grains can help resolve inflammatory processes by helping to achieve weight loss and by nourishing valuable gut bacteria linked with lower levels of inflammation. What we eat can make a difference in the inflammation associated with arthritis.

Types of Anti-inflammatory Foods to Eat to Help Arthritis

Foods Rich in Omega-3: Wild-caught fish, including salmon, is your best choice for omega-3 fats. Other foods to include in your diet include chia seeds, flax seeds, grass-fed beef, and walnuts.

Foods Rich in Sulfur: Sulfur boosts antioxidants and can help repair joints. Foods rich in sulfur include broccoli, brussels sprouts, cabbage, cauliflower, chives, collard greens, garlic, onions, garlic, grass-fed beef, leeks, organic eggs, radishes, raw dairy, watercress and wild-caught fish.

Bone Broth: Bone broth also makes the list for your arthritis diet because of its remarkable healing properties. According to nutrition researchers from the Weston A. Price Foundation, bone broth contains chondroitin sulfates and glucosamine which are the very compounds available in costly supplements designed to decrease joint pain and inflammation.

Fruits and Vegetables: Like every anti-inflammatory diet, fruits and vegetables are an important component. They provide digestive enzymes as well as anti-inflammatory compounds. When it comes to arthritis two of the best to be sure to include in your diet are papaya, which contains papain, and pineapple, which contains bromelain which research has shown may aid in decreasing disease-causing inflammation with ailments like rheumatoid arthritis.

Chapter 9: Anti-Inflammatory Herbs

Chronic inflammation is long-term. It results from the failure to eliminate whatever is causing the original acute inflammation and can last for months or even years. When people have inflammation, it often results in pain because of biochemical progressions that occur during inflammation leading to swelling that presses against sensitive nerve endings. This influences how nerves behave and can enhance pain. As a result, the kind of pain varies from one person to another and might come in the form of stiffness, discomfort, and even agony, but the thing sufferers have in common is that the pain is constant. It might be described as steady throbbing, stabbing, or pinching. Symptoms of chronic inflammation present in a number of ways including abdominal pain, chest pain, fatigue, fever, joint pain, mouth sores, muscle weakness and sometimes pain, and rashes.

Because of the side effects associated with traditional painkillers, many are turning to more natural herbal methods for healing and pain management. We've mentioned a handful of herbs and herbal supplements in earlier chapters, but here we dedicate the entire chapter to anti-inflammatory herbs. However, before you include herbal supplements in your health regime, it is best to talk with your doctor or pharmacist regarding any possible interactions with prescription or over-the-counter medications you may be taking.

Cayenne pepper:

The health benefits of cayenne and other hot chili peppers have been recognized since ancient times. Natural compounds called capsaicinoids are found in cayenne and all chili peppers. It's what gives them their spice and anti-inflammatory properties.

Black pepper:

The sharp taste of black pepper makes it one of the most popular spices in the world, but the piperine compound that gives black pepper that taste so many love is also a compound that prevents inflammation and makes it effective in reducing symptoms of arthritis.

Cinnamon:

Cinnamon is a common but popular spice often used to add flavor baked treats, but studies have shown it offers so much more than good flavor. This spice is rich in antioxidants, helps the body fight infection, and has anti-inflammatory properties which can ease swelling and repair tissue damage. Sprinkle it in your coffee or tea for a touch of flavor as just one way to enjoy its healing benefits.

Cloves:

Cloves are a pungent spice known for its anti-inflammatory properties. Researchers at the University of Florida conducted a study that had participants consume cloves daily and found that in just seven days it significantly lowered one specific pro-inflammatory cytokine. Because of its strong flavor, cloves pair well with nutmeg and cinnamon to add a tasty kick to stews and means. It's also a popular addition to Indian cuisine.

Devil's Claw:

This herb originally comes from South Africa and has been a remedy for African and European traditional and folk doctors used for centuries to treat digestive problems, relieve pain, reduce fever, and to treat some pregnancy symptoms. It also goes by the names wood spider or the grapple plant and it makes a popular choice for people suffering from arthritis and other forms of joint or back pain when combined with bromelain. In supplement form, devil's claw is derived from the dried roots of the plant.

Research has shown it may have anti-inflammatory properties.

Ginger:

We talked about ginger as a supplement in chapter 5, but garlic in its natural form has been used for hundreds of years to treat things like constipation, sinus congestion, indigestion, colic and other digestive problems, as well as rheumatoid arthritis pain. When taken orally, garlic is said to be beneficial for helping with pain and arthritis. Cloves can be eaten raw or cooked, or it can be purchased as a supplement in powdered form in capsules or tablets. It's also available in liquid extracts and oils.

Rosemary:

Rosemary leaves are often used in cooking, but this herb is much more than an aromatic plant. It provides a whole range of possible health benefits. It's plentiful in antioxidants and anti-inflammatory compounds believed to aid in boosting the immune system.

Sage:

The medicinal use of sage goes way back. In the past, it's been used for ailments ranging from mental disorders to intestinal and digestive discomfort. In more recent years, studies show the health benefits of sage have grown since then. Not it appears to contain a range of anti-inflammatory and antioxidant compounds and research has reinforced some of its medical applications. Along with use in cooking, it is commonly used to make sage tea as a way to enjoy its many benefits.

Spirulina:

Spirulina is a blue-green algae and considered a superfood. It's a rich source of vitamin B12, full of antioxidants, and is approximately 62% amino acids. Research has established that Spirulina prevents the production and release of histamine, which is a chemical that kindles an inflammatory response in the body. Additional research confirms that Spirulina may lessen arthritis. However, Spirulina is not recommended for those who suffer from digestive issues because it is very difficult to digest.

Chapter 10: Start Feeling Better Instantly

Since we've covered how inflammation works, the health problems surrounding chronic inflammation, and the foods to eat to combat those problems, in this chapter we will discuss the benefits associated with eating a more plant-based diet along with other lifestyle aspects needed to help fight your way back to good health.

Growing evidence shows diet and lifestyle can either generate a pro-inflammatory environment or an anti-inflammatory environment. So, if you are suffering from chronic inflammation you can quickly start feeling better than you do at this moment by making lifestyle changes right now. The first step in is to start choosing the right foods, but it's more than that. Buying the right foods won't make a difference if you don't prepare them correctly. For that reason, it's just as important to learn how to prepare those foods using anti-inflammatory cooking methods (see chapter 6). If you don't, you can undo the very healthy benefits you're hoping to enjoy.

Remember, your daily food selections are the source of your chronic inflammation. To jumpstart your anti-inflammatory diet, embrace a more plant-based diet because when it comes to fighting chronic inflammation, one of the biggest benefits of consuming a plant-based diet is its ability to lower chronic inflammation levels. In fact, it is suggested that inflammation might just be the biggest reason why plant-based diets have been shown to promote health while our typical American diet promotes disease. To be clear, "plant-based" doesn't necessarily me no meat, because it can allow for limited quantities of fish and lean meat. What it does mean is a diet heavy in nutrient-dense vegetables and fruits that can aid in warding off inflammation and disease. In 2014 study on diet and inflammatory bowel disease, 33% of the participants in the study opted not to go with the proposed anti-inflammatory diet. The participants who did decide to follow the anti-inflammatory diet experienced enough relief that they could discontinue at least one of their medications.

Nutrient dense foods offer high levels of vitamins, minerals, and/or protein per serving. If you want to jumpstart your anti-inflammatory diet to start feeling better faster, along with buying and preparing nutrient-dense foods and preparing them properly, it's also important to stay hydrated, but to keep costs down your should drink tap water instead of bottled - unless you cannot drink the tap water in your area. Avoid chlorinated, waters because you're working to eliminate substances you don't need in your body. Staying hydrated helps to suppress cellular inflammation and will decrease inflammation in the body.

Along with taking care of what you put into your body, it's also important that you get regular adequate exercise. Doing so can actually boost your immune system. Not being active enough is actually hard on your body, but be careful to not overdo it. Plan 20-30 minutes of light to moderate exercise most day. With physical activity comes free radical damage and the breaking down of body tissue. This results in some low-level inflammation in the body as it heals during the recovery time between active times. So the goal is to find the middle ground. To be active, but not overactive. To move enough, but to rest enough. If you don't do this, it can result in inflammation to build up.

As the repairing and restoring process works within the body while you sleep, it's hard at work. For this reason, getting enough rest is important with doctors recommending 7 to 8 hours of sleep per night. If you're lacking in sleep, you're taking advantage of your immune system. As a result, it needs to work harder to try to keep you well. Lack of sleep leads to stress. Constant stress produces more cortisol and you guessed it, inflammation.

Jason Michaels

So as you work to eat right, you need to put in the effort to also be active enough and to get your rest. It really is a lifestyle.

Chapter 11: Anti-inflammatory Meal Plan for 1 Week

As you reach toward better health going forward, your new goal is to consume a variety of nutrient-dense whole foods that can reduce inflammation. Making this move doesn't have to be hard, and it doesn't have to be expensive. You have plenty of foods to choose from and when you buy fruits and vegetable in season you will often find they cost less than a dollar per serving. The following list offers examples of anti-inflammatory foods that cost under a dollar per serving using in-season produce prices.

- Apples: $0.75 each
- Broccoli: $0.50 per 1/2 cup, $1.99 per bunch
- Cage-free Eggs: $0.25 per egg based on $2.99 a dozen
- Canned salmon: $0.80 for 4 oz. serving, based on $2.50 for 14.75 oz. can
- Cantaloupe: $0.50 for 1/2 cup, $3 per small melon and in season you can find them for much less
- Carrots: $0.50 each at $2 per pound
- Chicken breast: $0.75 for a 4-ounce serving, $2.99 per pound
- Garlic: $0.30 per bulb

Jason Michaels

- Grapes: $0.75 per cup, $1.50 per pound
- Kiwi: $0.40 each
- Mandarin oranges: $0.23 per piece, $3.99 for 5 pounds
- Onions: $0.18 each, $0.59 per pound
- Whole grain oats: $0.13 per serving, $3.98 for 30 oz. container. You can find oats for even less if you buy in bulk.

When you stop and really consider how many servings you get for your money when buying healthy foods, cost shouldn't really be a deterrent.

Sample Meal Plan for One Week

Day 1
Breakfast: Scrambled eggs served with chopped cabbage and onions seasoned with cumin seeds and turmeric. Steam until cabbage is softened but lightly crisp.
Lunch: Grilled salmon served on a bed of spring greens with olive oil and vinegar.
Dinner: Chicken breast seasoned with fresh herbs, and zesty lemon, steamed broccoli, and a serving of steamed brown rice.
Snack: 1 cup frozen grapes

Day 2

Breakfast: Oats (high in fiber, low in fat, oats contain avenanthramides which play a role in reducing inflammation). Add fruit like sliced banana or fresh dark-colored berries and a handful of walnuts.

Lunch: Spiced lentil soup seasoned with cinnamon, cayenne pepper, cumin, turmeric, and cayenne pepper

Dinner: Salmon patty (made using canned salmon, eggs, garlic, shallot, ginger, coconut flour, walnuts, cumin, turmeric, salt, and pepper), garden salad, topped with your favorite anti-inflammatory dressing.

Snack: Turmeric Chai Chia Pudding (from The Blenderist)

Day 3

Breakfast: Poached eggs served on fat-free refried beans topped with fresh salsa with sliced avocado on the side.

Lunch: Blueberry Banana smoothie made with coconut water and frozen banana

Dinner: Chicken curry made with sweet potato, broccoli, and cauliflower

Snack: Cup of diced cantaloupe

Day 4

Breakfast: Savory oats seasoned with cinnamon, a touch of ground coriander, ground cloves, ground ginger, a sprinkle of nutmeg and ground cardamom. Drizzle with a little real maple syrup which has a molecule with anti-inflammatory properties.

Lunch: Roasted sweet potato cut into strips like fries and served with avocado dip for a surprisingly delicious pairing

Dinner: Roasted garlic salmon with steamed cauliflower

Snack: Bell pepper strips with guacamole

Day 5

Breakfast: Pineapple smoothie made with green tea, kale, pineapple, frozen mango chunks, a tsp. of fresh ginger, and a pinch of turmeric

Lunch: Roasted red pepper and sweet potato soup

Dinner: Baked cod with pecan rosemary topping, and steamed green beans,

Snack: Cup of cherries

Day 6

Breakfast: Spinach and mushroom frittata

Lunch: Fruit salad made from your favorite in-season fruits

Dinner: Bell peppers, mushrooms, onions and diced tomatoes with chicken breast chunks, season with cayenne pepper for a little zip. Serve with quinoa

Snack: Dark chocolate

Day 7

Breakfast: Oatmeal seasoned with turmeric topped with plenty of colorful berries. Unique but delicious.

Lunch: Miso soup with gluten-free noodles

Dinner: Turkey and quinoa stuffed bell peppers

Snack: A serving of almonds

Conclusion

Thanks for making reading Anti-Inflammatory Diet: Make these simple, inexpensive changes to your diet and start feeling better within 24 hours!, let's hope it was informative and able to provide you with all of the tools you need to achieve your goals whatever they may be.

If the effects of chronic inflammation are robbing you of the joy of living because of pain, fatigue, weight gain or other health issues, it's time to take charge of your health. Now that you've read this book you are equipped to take steps toward healing. You've seen the statistics. Embrace the hope found in these pages and be proactive. Set a goal to consume less processed and fast foods and more fresh foods plentiful in fruits and vegetables. If you really want to see improvement, focus on health and healing, and that means thinking about every bite of food you take to get to your goal.

Don't be afraid to give up those favorite processed foods. They might taste good, but think about what you're really eating. Things like inflammation-triggering preservatives, artificial flavorings, and colorings, and then ask yourself if you want to still eat them. Don't think of it as depriving yourself, but instead think of it as empowering yourself to live healthier and pain-free. You don't have to be a slave to foods that aren't good for you, and you don't have to be controlled by pain or poor health.

Enjoy a piece of chocolate, and a cup of coffee and feel guilt free as you learn to eliminate inflammation triggering foods from your diet. You'll find a sense of freedom in just feeling better. Yes, it can take time, but remember it took time for the inflammation your fighting to become chronic. Each day is worth the fight toward better health, and now you have the arsenal at your fingertips to fight it.

Finally, if you found this book useful in any way, a review on Amazon is always appreciated!

Yours in health,
Jason Michaels

Intermittent Fasting for Beginners

The Proven Way to Lose Weight,

Build Muscle and Live a Healthy,

Food-Stress-Free Lifestyle

By

Jason Michaels

Introduction

Congratulations on downloading *"Intermittent Fasting for Beginners: The Proven Way to Lose Weight, Build Muscle and Live a Healthy Lifestyle."* Thank you for doing so.

The food pyramid model for eating was first introduced in Sweden in 1974 and spread throughout other Scandinavian countries, Sri Lanka and West Germany. The food pyramid was introduced to the United States in 1992 and was replaced by MyPlate in 2011 after people realized the pyramid was terribly erroneous. The model's focus on heavy carbohydrate intake contributed to making the citizens of the United States among the world's largest populations of obese people.

At the same time, the quick-paced, modern lifestyle also contributed to poor eating habits. Fast food, with its emphasis on cheap starchy and sugary food, replaced many healthy homemade meals.

According to the World Health Organization, as of 2014 more than 1.9 billion adults over the age of 18 were overweight worldwide, and 600 million of those would be considered obese. Additionally, 41 million children younger than 5 were considered overweight or obese.

However, a recent movement toward natural eating brought a resurgence in various popular diets and eating habits that resemble those of our ancestors. One of these diets involves the practice of intermittent fasting.

The following chapters describe what fasting is, the science behind fasting, and why meal timing is irrelevant. The various intermittent fasting structures are explained, as well as how to use intermittent fasting to lose weight or to build muscles. This book also gives specific information about meal plans, eating schedules, and exercising.

There are plenty of books on this subject on the market. Thanks again for choosing this one! Every effort was made to ensure it is full of as much useful information as possible. Good luck in your journey toward a thinner, healthier you!

Chapter 1: What is Fasting?

There are a number of different definitions as to how long between meals, or what intake determines a fast. Fasting can be summarized as the deliberate act of not eating or drinking for a period of time.

Sometimes a person drinks juice ("juice fasting") or water but does not eat. This can be considered a fast depending on your diet plan.

Technically, we all fast daily if we get eight hours of sleep every night. If we also don't eat several hours before bedtime, or if we skip breakfast, we have had a mini-fast of 12 hours. It's that easy.

"Intermittent fasting" is when a person skips at least one meal, then eats, then fasts, and so on. A person is considered to have entered a period of fasting if they have not eaten for more than eight hours.

Fasting is not a new phenomenon however. Humans have been fasting for thousands of years. Historically, people fasted for various reasons, not just limited to health. These included religious and medical reasons.

Jason Michaels

Fasting in History: Religious reasons

When fasting is done for religious reasons, it is sometimes viewed as a symbolic gesture that serves to teach people to not be selfish or act upon carnal desires. Various religions also consider fasting to aid in meditation. Thus, religious leaders often tell parishioners to engage in "fasting and prayer."

Buddhist monks and nuns fast daily after their noon meals until the next morning. They think of this practice as something that aids in meditation and contributes to good health, however, they do not consider this daily practice to be fasting. Buddhists consider long-term periods of eating very little food to be fasting by their traditional definition, and they fast in this sense when they want to practice intense meditation.

Many members of Christianity embrace the practice of fasting because of various Bible passages, such as Isaiah 58:6-7, which was written to the Israelites and spoke of an "acceptable fast." This had to do with following all commandments.
Fasting is practiced in some, but not all denominations of Christianity.

Those that do engage in this practice include both Pentecostals and Charismatics as the result of individual choice, but the Charismatics commonly choose to do it once weekly.

The Eastern Orthodox Church and the Catholic Church practice a forty-day partial fast every year. The Eastern Orthodox Church considers fasting as part of a connection between body and the soul. The Ethiopian Orthodox Church does not eat meat or consume milk in any form for several weeks, several times every year.

Roman Catholics have strict fasting rules for parishioners who are between the ages of 18 and 59 during Lent. The Anglican Church also has strict fasting rules, as do the Assyrian Church of the East. Lutheran and Reformed churches take a much less stringent position on fasting.

The Church of Jesus Christ of Latter Day Saints, better known as the Mormons fast two meals on the first Sunday of every month, and the money saved by not eating is donated to the church. Hindus fast on particular day of the month.

Jason Michaels

This historical practice demonstrates that the act of fasting is one that is more than just a passing health fad, and more so an act deep seated across societies worldwide.

Fasting for medical reasons

Patients are required to abstain from eating food before their blood, cholesterol, or glucose levels are tested and before they are screened for diabetes. That is because food can interfere with test results. A partial fast that only allows clear liquids to be consumed is required just before a colonoscopy.

Patients must not eat before having a major surgery that involves the use of anesthesia. If a patient eats just before surgery, he could vomit, inhale the vomit and die while he is unconscious. Regurgitation while under anesthesia is rare, however, so fasting may no longer be required of surgery patients in the near future.

Fasting for health reasons

There are several benefits of intermittent fasting over other weight loss methods.

Detoxification - One benefit is the fact that fasting causes the body to detoxify. Toxic buildup occurs because of a poor diet and because of eating frequently (meals eaten less than six hours apart). The body needs to take a break from processing food so that it can cleanse the digestive tract.

Weight Loss - When people fast, the body helps them lose weight in two ways. Most people carry between five and twenty pounds of food in their intestines. When a person fasts, their body gets rid of much of the impacted feces on its own, although drinking sea salt in warm water or senna tea while fasting helps tremendously. Old waste matter is one source of the extra weight.

Not including water retention, the other source of extra weight is, of course, fat. When the body does not receive food within about 12 hours, it starts to use stored-up fat for fuel.

Hunger Management - Another benefit of intermittent fasting is hunger management. When you are not fasting, your blood sugar level decreases and your brain receives a message that you are hungry. When you fast intermittently, however, your body burns the fat and the hunger hormones are turned off. This allows our bodies to reduce the feeling of hunger and we are less likely to be struck by food cravings that are prone to throw us off our diets.

Reduced Risk of Type II Diabetes - Since intermittent fasting causes your body to burn all of the glucose in your body before it burns fat for energy, your blood sugar levels remain low. Low blood sugar levels decrease the risk of getting Type II diabetes. A 2009 study published by the *Scandanvian Journal of Clinical and Laboratory Investigation* found that intermittent fasting resulted in a 3 to 6% reduction of blood sugar that caused a 20 to 31% reduction in insulin. Intermittent fasting also increases the dieter's sensitivity to insulin.

Slowing Down of the Aging Process - The lowering of blood sugar that happens during intermittent fasting forces the body's cells to remove unhealthy mitochondria, which reduces production of free radicals. When there are less free radicals, there is less oxidative stress which leads to a slowing down of the aging process.

Reduced Risk of Cancer – Whether or not intermittent fasting reduces the risk of cancer is a topic that continues to be heavily debated, but it is thought to at least be effective against breast cancer. However, one study performed by USC's D. Valter Longo and reported in the research journal *Cell Metabolism* that was done on 10 cancer patients demonstrated that intermittent fasting caused the fasting patients to respond better to the chemotherapy and to have better cure rates than cancer patients who did not fast. Cancer results from uncontrolled growth of cells, and those cells rely on glucose to grow. That is why less food would logically slow down the growth of cancer cells.

Longevity – Cell Metabolism also reported on numerous studies on rats demonstrated that intermittent fasting caused the rats to live 83% longer than the rats that were fed regularly.

Other anecdoctal eveidence - Various conditions alleviated by fasting, including constipation, stomach problems, addictions, rheumatic conditions, arthritis, asthma, heart disease, high blood pressure, high cholesterol levels, poor pancreas performance, sleep problems, mood swings, and mild depression. People have reported experiencing an increase in energy, clarity of mind, an increase in sex drive, a feeling of being clean inside, and a sense of overall well-being after they fast.

Jason Michaels

Chapter 2: The Science Behind Intermittent Fasting

A General Understanding

When a person eats regularly, the body breaks down the food that is eaten into glucose. Glucose triggers the production of insulin. Insulin helps the body use the glucose for energy and stores the unused glucose as fat because the fat is not used for energy.

After 12 hours of fasting, the body starts to burn fat, the body is forced to burn the stored fat because there is no glucose left to use for fuel. This is when weight loss happens. This is also the most effective time to exercise.

As fasting is most often thought of as not consuming calories at all for a period of time. Intermittent fasting is fasting for a short while and then starting back up with eating, cycling back and forth between eating and not eating.

Ancient man hunted for food after he went without food for several hours. This was not by choice, he fasted intermittently on a daily basis due to a lack of consistent food supply (and convenience stores!). Intermittent fasting brought about optimum and constant burning of fat for fuel rather than glucose. This was compounded by consuming only natural, healthy food. The hard life they led forced them into a healthy way of eating.

General calorie restriction is undernourishment without malnourishment, so as long as a person is not undernourished for long periods of time and he eats quality food when he eats, his body does not suffer from any health based consequences.

Clinical Studies

Many studies have been done on the effects of calorie restriction (low-calorie diets) on the health of humans and animals, but the effects of intermittent fasting on humans where no food is allowed occasionally has not been widely clinically studied.

One study that was performed by Martin, Mattson and Maudsley (of the United States National Institutes of Health) in 2006 and reported by the journal *Aging Research Reviews* indicated that the effects of intermittent fasting on health are similar to those of low-calorie diets.

Both calorie restriction and intermittent fasting put stress on cells, which brings about resistance to metabolic and environmental stress without doing any harm.
Calorie restriction and intermittent fasting also increase insulin sensitivity and reduce glucose and insulin levels.

Intermittent fasting studies performed on animals by Mark Mattson, senior investigator for the National Institute on Aging, showed that the test subjects who were subjected to intermittent fasting experienced better learning abilities, memory, reduced oxidative stress, and showed improvement in diseases.

Studies performed on humans showed that the body goes to fat stores for energy after 10 to 16 hours of fasting. Not surprisingly, the studies also showed that the body starts to quickly bring down a person's weight when a person combines intermittent fasting with a low-calorie diet that consists of quality food.

Mattson thought that perhaps the body resists disease because fasting puts the body's cells under mild stress, which brings about adaptation from the stress. This is what the body does when a person exercises.

Chapter 3: Why Meal Timing is Irrelevant for Weight Loss & Muscle Gain

You will notice that the timing of the meals eaten in each of the various intermittent fasting diet plans is different from that of the others, and yet all of these intermittent fasting plans work. For example, one diet has you not eating for an entire 24 hours, while others have you eating every day, but within smaller windows of time.

Time of Day

The time of day that you eat meals is irrelevant due to two main factors.

First of all, you will restrict the overall calorie count for each week while you are fasting intermittently, which means that you will burn more calories than you consume, no matter what time of day that you eat or drink those calories. This is the first law of thermodynamics and the basic science behind all diets or weight loss plans.

Granted, if you eat earlier in the day, you have time to burn the glucose, but any time you burn more calories than you eat and drink, you lose weight. Any additional exercise will also burn calories.

Secondly, you will burn fat instead of glucose around the clock when you fast intermittently. The time of day that you eat will not change that fact either.

Other diet plans may have you timing your carbohydrate intake. With intermittent fasting, this is no longer an issue. So long as you are at a net calorie deficit at the end of the day/week, the timing of eating carbs is not a big issue to the intermittent faster. You could only have carbs just before you work out in the gym so that you would have energy during that time. Contrary to that would be a program like the warrior diet which allows you to eat some carbs late at night when you do all of your eating for the day. This diet is ideal for gaining muscle weight and tends to be favored by bodybuilders who fast intermittently.

Eating carbohydrates in the morning is the kind of thing that we are used to when we are eating on a regular 3 meals a day schedule. However, 3 square meals a day has only been the societal norm for the past 300 years. Beforehand most advanced societies ate once or two daily. In fact, Yale University professor and editor of Food: The

History of Taste states "There is no biological reason for eating three meals a day."

If you eat bread, pasta, etc., and do not fast, of course, it would be wise to eat carbohydrates in the morning so that you would have all day to burn off the large amount of glucose that will form in your body. Otherwise, the insulin would make all of that glucose convert to fat if you did not burn the required calories.

People argue that those of us who skip breakfast are fatter than people who eat breakfast, yet there is no data to back up this claim. They also claim that muscles will fall off if one is following an IF protocol. But the human metabolism does not change that quickly, which studies in both intermittent fasting and general fasting have shown.

In fact, the metabolic rate rises abruptly during the first 72 hours that a person fasts, and it takes the body between three and four days before a fast or a strict partial fast negatively affects metabolism. The idea that skipping one meal here and there affects metabolism, therefore, is erroneous.

Meal Frequency

Jason Michaels

When it comes to weight loss, there is much literature regarding "stoking the metabolic fire" if you were to eat six times per day and that skipping just one meal per day would slow down your metabolism.

This concept came from a misunderstanding of dietary-induced thermogenesis (DIT), which deals with how many calories the body burns while digesting food.

In the studies that were conducted which led to this notion that people need to eat frequently, the subject's metabolism was increasing because people ate more food during the day, not because they ate frequently.

If the study participants eating six meals per day ate the same number of calories daily as people who ate only three times per day did, there would have been no difference in the DIT. For example, six meals of 300 calories is the same total caloric intake as three meals of 600 calories.

What the participants did, though, was to eat more calories when they ate six times daily. Eating more food to raise metabolism is like being excited to save $100 by spending $800. It looks good on paper - but in actual terms, it just doesn't make sense.

From a practical standpoint, a smaller person needing a lower calorie intake on a diet where several small meals are required throughout the day would literally be eating a couple of bites of things at every meal if he or she were to stay within their calorie limit. So more meals for small people often does not make much practical sense, this is especially true for females.

The number of times that you eat in a day does not matter when it comes to retaining lean muscle tissue either, just as long as the daily intake of protein is high. Meal frequency only negatively affects lean muscles if the meal frequency promotes food choices that offer inadequate level of proteins to maintain muscle mass which is about 0.8g per lb of muscle mass over the course of a day.

Not only are low-sugar protein shakes effective sources of protein that will enable you to keep or build muscles, but these shakes also fill you up quickly and are low-calorie.

Chapter 4: The Various Intermittent Fasting Structures

16/8 Method

Best for: **People who will frequently work out in a gym, building muscles and losing fat.**

Creator: **This method was formulated by personal trainer and nutritional expert, Martin Berkhan**

How it Works: This diet is very simple. The dieter fasts for 16 hours per day if a man (14 hours per day if you are a woman) and eats within the remaining hours.

It does not matter which hours of the day that you choose, but as with all IF protocols you would likely want to schedule your fasting time around your sleeping hours.

If you do not work a first-shift job, the suggested way to schedule these daily fasts is to start your fast just after you eat dinner, sleep, exercise throughout the morning, and break your fast (at "breakfast") after you have fasted the 16 or 14 hours.

You can eat more carbohydrates on the days that you work out than on the days that you don't work out. On days that you do not work out, you need to consume more dietary fat.

Protein intake should be high every day, but even that depends on the amount of body fat that you have, your general activity level, your gender, age, goals, etc. As with all diets, keep processed food intake to a minimum. Protein shakes that contain fruit and vegetables in addition to the protein powder are acceptable as meal replacements, as are protein meal replacement bars (though in moderation, as many of these contain high levels of sugar).

If you follow this schedule, the only time you might feel a little hungry would be in the morning. If you are not working out, drink water, black coffee, unsweetened tea, or green tea during these late hours in your fast. If you put lemon in your water, you will further suppress the hunger. The caffeine in both coffee and tea increase the intensity of the fat burning that is occurring during these hours in addition to suppressing hunger.

Green tea suppresses hunger, burns fat, and also increases your metabolism. It increases metabolism because it has various bioactive properties such as EGCG as well as the

Jason Michaels

aforementioned caffeine. These agents also interact with your hormones to better break down the fat.

Using this plan, the most effective time to work out is on an empty stomach. Working out while you are hungry doesn't sound like an attractive plan, but there is a way to get around that. This answer is drinking BCAA protein shake just before you work out.

Assuming you are doing this in the morning, you can then break your fast by eating something. If you like to work out in the evening, schedule your workout one or two hours after you have eaten.

Pros: People find this diet attractive because the timing and the frequency of meals is fairly flexible on the days that you don't work out, although most people still break up their eating into three meals.

Cons: This diet has strict guidelines as to what food you can eat, especially when it comes to your workout days. Some people find it hard to stick to the program because of this inflexibility.

EatStopEat

Best for: **People who already eat healthy and are just needing a little boost.**

Creator: **This method was created by Brad Pilon, who had a background in nutrition and in the sports supplement industry. He created it based on the fact that brief, regular fasts help people to lose weight while retaining muscle mass.**

How it Works: On this diet, the dieter does not eat for 24 hours one or two days per week. He or she can have calorie-free drinks (no milk or sugar) during the fasting days and then eat as they normally eat during the other days.

The rationale is simply to cut out overall calories taken in, however, doing a small amount of resistance training during just three of the days that you eat is key to losing weight and improving your overall body composition. Just simple compound exercises focusing on full body training (squats, deadlifts, bench press) during those three days will make the difference. Exercising on days that you eat sets this plan apart from some of the other plans that require you to work out on an empty stomach.

Jason Michaels

Start this fast after dinner one day and break it at dinner the next day, having only skipped breakfast and lunch. If you are new to fasting, you should fast just one day per week in the beginning. In time, you can increase this to fast two days per week. If even one day proves to be too difficult, start with just a 15-hour fast and add another hour with each fast that you do. Start a fast on a day that you will be naturally busy or when you are not scheduled to eat with other people.

Some people schedule a fast just before they attend a party because they can break their fast eating the party food (in moderation) without feeling guilty. It is best to not eat any junk food. But if you will attend a party anyway, this is one way to not lose any ground where your weight is concerned.

Pros: This plan is flexible. If you can't go without food for 24 hours, you can start with just 15 hours and work your way up as your body adjusts to fasting. Another good thing about this diet is that you do not count calories, weigh food, or restrict your diet (other than avoiding a free-for-all, junk food diet). Also, this diet retains lean muscle tissue better than the other methods do.

Cons: People can suffer headaches, fatigue, foul moods, or anxiety when they suddenly go without food for 24 hours. People also tend to binge-eat when they come off of this fast, finding self-control hard when they are hungry.

The Warrior Diet

Best for: **Disciplined, devoted people who can follow rules.**

Creator: **This plan was formulated by fitness expert, Ori Hofmekler, who studied how the lean and muscular ancient Romans and Spartans ate.**

How it Works: **The ancient Romans and Spartans ate very little during the day and then feasted on food they hunted during the evenings. If body building is your thing, this should be your intermittent fasting diet of choice.**

This diet is similar to the Martin Berghan's diet except you eat very small portions of food for 20 hours every day and then eat a lot of food during a period of just four hours every evening.

Even this diet needs to be eased into because the dieter can experience the same symptoms of hunger as if they didn't eat anything at all for all of those hours.

In your first week, skip breakfast once or twice a week. Skip breakfast three or four times the next week. Move into skipping lunch and work on up to skipping all breakfasts and lunches every day.

You may nibble on raw fruits and vegetables, eat small amounts of protein, and drink fresh juice during the days. This maximizes the "fight or flight" response from the sympathetic nervous system. This response promotes alertness, boosts energy, and burns fat.

When you break your fast at night, you must eat particular food groups in a particular order. First, you eat broth, then vegetables, protein/meat, and then fat. You can eat carbohydrates at the end of your four-hour feasting period if you are still hungry.

Eating at night maximizes the parasympathetic nervous system, which helps the body to recuperate, become calm, relax, digest while the body uses the nutrients for growth and for repair. It may also help the body to produce fat-burning hormones that work on your fat the next day.

Another aspect of this diet is to do strength training during the daytime. Do squats, pull-ups, high jumps, press-ups, frog jumps and sprints. Select three of these activities, doing two sets of five minutes each during a thirty-minute period of time that you set aside every day. Drink a protein shake before you exercise.

Pros: A person who can regularly follow this diet will turn his or her body into a fat-burning and muscle-forming machine! One also gets to eat something during the fasting time, which helps the person endure the fasting hours. People experience increased energy and greater loss of fat when they adopt this eating style.

Cons: The strict schedule and eating guidelines are hard for some people to follow, especially if they have to attend a lot of social gatherings. Additionally, some people prefer to not eat large meals late at night.

Alternate Day Fasting

Best for: **Disciplined people who have a weight goal in mind.**

Jason Michaels

Creator: **This diet was formulated by Dr. James Johnson especially for goal-minded disciplined dieters.**

How it Works: Of the two intermittent fasting diets that mainly have weight loss in mind, this one is better optimized for your end goal.

On this diet, the dieter does a partial fast every other day, eating a limited amount of food for one day and then a normal amount the next day, and so on.

Because there are seven days in the week and the diet follows a schedule by the week day, the dieter uses three specific days of every week to do a partial fast. Dieters using this model commonly choose to diet on Mondays, Wednesdays, and Fridays.

On those days, the dieter consumes only one-fifth of the normal number of calories that he or she consumes on the other days. If you are a man, you likely take in about 2,500 calories per day. If you are a woman, you likely consume about 2,000 calories per day. Therefore, you would consume 500 or 400 calories on Mondays, Wednesdays, and Fridays, which can easily be done by drinking protein shakes.

Protein shakes are very filling and are also low in calories. High-protein foods and vegetables will also help you to fill up faster. The experts sometimes recommend protein shakes for just the first two weeks of the diet and real food from the third week onward.

Working out is not advised on this program, If you must work out while on this diet, do a lighter version of your regular workouts on the days that you eat normally.

Pros: This diet can effectively drop about 2.5 pounds of weight per week for dieters who cut their calorie intake between 20 and 35 percent, and this is done without the dieter feeling hungry or having to follow a difficult schedule. Additionally, dieting on alternate days never allows leptin levels to fall, which means that the body never stops losing the fat.

Cons: The dieter must be careful to not binge eat on their off days. This is not a program aimed for beginners or those who only need a slight reduction in weight.

The 5:2 Diet

Best for: People who are not sensitive to blood sugar levels.

Creator: This diet became popular because of the work of Dr. Michael Mosley, who was also a journalist.

How it Works: In this diet, you eat normally for five days of the week and reduce your calorie intake for two days of the week that are not consecutive days. Decide on the two days of the week you will diet and diet on those days every week.

When you eat normally, the calorie count needs to be 2,500 for men and 2,000 for women. On the partial fasting days, your calories should be 600 for men and 500 for women. You also consume those calories in two meals on fasting days, with 300 calories per meal for men and 250 calories per meal for women.

Green smoothies made of zucchini, celery, broccoli, lentils, kales, collards, mustard, and spinach are low in calories and will fill you up fast. Watermelon and broth-based soups will also fill you up fast. Drink a lot of water on the partial fasting days.

Pros: The plan is easy. It is similar to the EatStopEat plan, but you fast (partially) just two days of the week.

Cons: This diet is not advisable for people who have a history of eating disorders, or are sensitive to fluctuations in blood sugar levels.

Chapter 5: Intermittent Fasting for Weight Loss

As you read in the previous chapter, programs exist for people whose goal is to lose the fat and not necessarily to build up muscle.

If weight loss is your main goal, you have a choice between the Alternate Day Fast or the 5:2 Diet if using intermittent fasting.

	Alternate Day Fast	**The 5:2 Diet**
Fasting schedule	Partially fast three full alternate days.	Partially fast two full alternate days.
Fasting time food/cal	Men=500; Wm=400 Vegetable soup, salad or other veggies with	Men=600; Wm=500 Divide calories between two meals. Green

chicken or turkey, eggs
(veggie-based) smoothies,
with veggies, and yogurt
watermelon, broth-based
with berries would be   soup
would be good
good options. Drink a
options. Drink a lot of
lot of water.
water.

Eat time food/cal   Men=2,500; Wm=2,000
Men=2,500; Wm=2,000
Normal food, little junk.
Normal food, little junk.

Missed meals   N/A   N/A

Exercise   None
None to very light

Restrictions   None   Wm
trying to conceive
          Wm
breastfeeding

Glucose-sensitive people

Have eating disorder

Pros   Effective; no hunger
        Easiest; no hunger

Cons   Temptation to binge   Not
avail. to all people

Chapter 6: Intermittent Fasting for Muscle Gain

If you want to gain muscle as you lose the fat, you can choose from the Leangains, EatStopEat, and the Warrior intermittent fasting plans.

	16/8 (Berghan)	EatStopEat	Warrior
Fasting sched.	Fast 16 hours daily. Many people start right after dinner to take advantage of sleep hours.	Full fast 24 hours one or two days weekly. Many people start right after dinner. The next meal is the next day. If	Fast 20 hours daily, feasting nightly. You will likely need to fast fewer hours when you start this dinnerdiet and work up to 20 hours. This diet

Jason Michaels

                              you cannot fast 24

tells you to eat at

                              hours, try to start

night, so start your

                              with 15 hours.

fast after your large

dinner.

Fast'g time food No calories *except* No calories.
Drink Munch on *small*

                10g protein before, water, coffee, tea,
amounts of raw

                10g protein 1 hour or green tea.
fruit and veggies,

                after finishing, and
protein food, just

                10g 2 hours later.
enough for energy.

                Also drink water,
Drink water, coffee,

                coffee, tea, or
tea, green tea, or

                green tea.
juice.

Eat time food	Eat anything in moderation.	Eat anything in moderation.
This diet dictates that you eat in this order: broth, veggies, meat or seafood, then carbs.	Limit junk food. Can have more carbs on days you exercise, which should be every day. Eat more healthy fats on days you don't exercise. Can substitute protein shakes or protein bars for meals.	Limit junk food.
Missed meals Two meals (partial fast), with a protein	One (though replaced with	Two meals

Jason Michaels

30g protein)
shake before exer-

cising.

Exercise Exercise 1 hour On *3 of your eat*
Do strength
  every morning, *days*, do 2 sets
training, such as
  preferably 12 for 3 reps of 3
squats, pull-ups,
  hours into your of the following
press-ups, high
  fast. You could exerises: leg
jumps, sprints,
  exercise evenings extensions,
dumb-frog jumps, etc.,
  2 hours after your bell lunges, seated
for 30 minutes
  last meal if you calf raises, seated
daily. Choose 3
  don't want to rows, pull-ups,
exercises, 2 sets
  exercise mornings. one-arm
dumbbell for 5 minutes

108

bar-	each.	preacher curl, Bell bench press-wide grip, push-ups with feet elevated, or front dumbbell raises.
Restrictions None	None	None
Pros This diet turns your body into a fat-burning, muscle-making machine! Some food is allowed during fasting	Flexible timing and frequency of meals on eat days.	Flexible number of diet hours. No calorie counting. No weighing food. No strict dietary restrictions on eat

times, which

helps people to

stay on the diet.

People experience

greater energy.

days. Retains

lean muscles

better than the

other methods.

Cons

Strict dietary
guidelines and
eating schedules
are hard for some
people to follow
all the time. Some

people don't like

to eat large meals

Strict dietary

guidelines, espe-

cially on fasting

days, are hard for

some people to

follow.

The long fasting

time causes foul

moods, fatigue,

headaches, and

anxiety on fasting

days. People

tend to binge eat

on eat days.

late at night.

Jason Michaels

Chapter 7: Intermittent Fasting and Exercise

Food is the fuel that your body uses to power itself and to build new muscle when exercising. With that in mind, it shouldn't be surprising that the timing of your meals can easily have a serious impact both on how easily you will find a given workout and also how effective that workout will be.

Adding exercise to an intermittent fasting plan

It doesn't matter if you are training for endurance or training to improve your strength, your body primarily uses the glycogen found in stored carbohydrates to fuel your exercise. However, when your glycogen reserves are running low, such as when you are in the latter half of a period of fasting, then your body is going to need to look to other energy sources like fat to power your exercise routine. This means that you are likely to burn up to 20 percent more fat if you exercise during a fast as opposed to just after you have broken one.

Unfortunately, it is not all good news as when glycogen is in short supply in your body, you are also more likely to burn protein as well as fat. As protein is what helps to build muscles, exercising in the midst of fast is likely to cause you to lose muscle mass as well. Depending on how much you plan on exercising and how long it has been since you have eaten any carbs, your body may start burning protein for energy as soon as you get started.

This won't just affect how much you can bench press or how toned your body looks, it will also slow your metabolism which will make it more difficult for you to lose weight in the long run as your body naturally adapts to the number of calories you are consuming on a regular basis over time. As such, once your body gets used to the fact that you are consuming fewer calories per day on average your body will eventually get used to burning fewer calories each day to ensure that you have enough energy left over for the basics such as staying healthy, breathing and even staying upright throughout the day. It will typically take about a month of regular rounds of fasting for your body to adapt to the change.

Finally, when planning on how to merge your exercise plan with an intermittent fasting lifestyle it is important to keep in mind that it is naturally going to be more difficult to exercise on an empty stomach. When your blood sugar and glycogen levels are low you are going to naturally feel weaker than you otherwise would. What's more, if you don't schedule your workouts at the end of a fast then your results will suffer as your body won't have the tools it needs to build muscle.

Intermittent fasting and exercise tips

Prioritize low-intensity cardio: If you plan on exercising regularly while you are fasting, it is important to limit your cardio to low-intensity options. This means you should still be able to carry on a conversation with relative ease if you are exercising during a fast. Ideally, you are going to want to stick to things like a light jog or 25 minutes on a cardio machine and be sure not to push yourself too hard. It will also be extra important to listen to your body and take a breather if you start to feel dizzy or light-headed which is going to happen much more often than it otherwise would. If you ignore this advice and push your exercise intensity level to the limit then it will make the rest of your workout feel like much more of a struggle regardless of what you are doing.

Choose your battles: This is not to say that you should never push your body to the limit while fasting. Instead, it is important to time your more intense periods of exercise to about an hour after you have eaten. This will give your body time to process the nutrients you have provided for it and will help you to maximize the amount of fat you can lose while still staying properly fueled for the workout by having plenty of glycogen in your system which will also help to reduce the risk of low blood sugar levels. Additionally, if you can afford to alter your fasting schedule slightly, following up a high-intensity workout with a snack that is high in carbs is also encouraged because your muscles will have burned through the available glycogen while still being hungry for more.

Up your protein intake: Standard workout convention suggest that you are going to want to take in between 20 and 30 grams of protein every four hours while you are awake. While intermittent fasting makes this unattainable, you're should still aim to take in between 80 and 120 grams of protein per day. If you are planning a serious strength workout then you should plan to do so between two snacks, if not two full meals.

Additionally, it is important to keep in mind that snacks are going to be your friend, as long as your intermittent fasting plan supports them, of course. A snack or a meal consumed between 3 and 4 hours before a workout should be enough to keep your blood sugar up through a standard workout, or between 1 and 2 hours if you are prone to low

Jason Michaels

blood sugar. These meals should include blood-sugar stabilizing protein along with fast-acting carbs, for example two pieces of whole wheat toast with banana slices and peanut butter. Additionally, sometime in the two hours after your workout you are going to want to try and consume approximately 20 grams of protein and 20 grams of carbs to ensure maximum muscle growth and to get your glycogen stores up high enough that you maintain energy until it is time to eat again.

Plan out your meals in the right way: Ideally you will want to be sure to consume a majority of your daily caloric intake in the period immediately following your workout period. This will not only make it easier for your body to generate lean muscle mass it will also make it easier to recover from the workout. In order to do this, you should start by determining the caloric requirements your body needs in order to build muscle.

To do so, you are going to need to determine your basal metabolic rate (BMR) which is the number of calories you burn while resting. The more lean muscle mass you have, the higher your BMR is going to be. Essentially what this means is that the more muscular physique you have, the more calories you are going to be burning around the clock.

The average human body burns about 60 percent of its daily calorie consumption just through natural daily processes. From there, the body burns about 30 percent of its energy on physical activity and 10 percent on digestion.

To determine how many calories your body burns while resting, you can use the following formula. First you will need to determine your weight in kilograms by dividing your current weight in pounds by 2.2. You will also need to determine your height in centimeters which can be found by taking your height in inches and multiplying by 2.54.

For men, your BMR will be equal to 66.47+(13.75 x weight in kilograms) + (5 x height in centimeters) − (6.75 x age).

For women, your BMR is going to be equal to (65.09 + (9.56 x weight in kilograms) + (1.84 x height in centimeters) − (4.67 x Age).

The end result is the number of calories you burn while your body is at rest. For example, for a man who weighs 200 lbs. their BMR would be about 2,200 calories. From there, you can use the Sterling-Pasmore Equation to determine how many calories you need based on your current amount of lean body mass. Each pound of lean muscle mass requires 13.8 calories to support it. You can determine your current lean body mass from standard body fat measurements.

Calculate lean muscle mass vs. fat mass:
Body fat % x scale weight= fat mass
Scale weight - fat mass= lean body mass

Once you have determined your BMR, you will want to account for the additional calories that are burned through exercise.

- If you live a primarily sedimentary lifestyle you will want to multiply your BMR by 1.2.
- If you perform a light exercise routine 3 or 4 times per week you you will want to multiply your BMR by 1.375.
- If you perform moderate exercise between 3 and 5 days per week you will want to multiply your BMR by 1.55
- If you exercise at a moderate intensity 6 or 7 days a week you will want to multiply your BMR by 1.725.
- If you are extremely active and exercise 6 or 7 days a week for 90 minutes or more you will want to multiply your BMR by 1.9 (this category is reserved for endurance athletes)

If you are not sure about your activity level, underestimate it rather than overestimate.

With your BMR in mind, you are then going to want to consume about 20 percent of those calories before you exercise for the best results. This meal or snack should be a quality mix of both carbs and protein. Then, when you are finished exercising you are going to want to consume about 60 percent of your total calories sometime in the next 2 to 4 hours. This might seem like a lot but if you focus on calorie dense foods it should not be a problem.

Additionally, with this type of setup it is important to keep in mind that you are typically better off focusing on a diet with more carbs and less fat to support muscle growth. This is due to the fact that, following a workout, you should focus on carb intake, instead of fats which can be detrimental. This doesn't mean you should eliminate all fats, it just means you are going to want to limit the number of fats you consume in your post-workout meals.

If you lead a mostly sedimentary lifestyle then you will want to take in about 31 calories per kilogram per day to maintain your weight. If you are a recreational athlete then this number will be between 33 and 38 calories. If you are an endurance athlete then this number will be between 35 and 50 calories based on your training. If you are strength training and exercising heavily then this will be between 30 and 60 calories based on your training.

If you are looking to build muscle mass then you should aim to ensure that you take in an additional 250 to 500 calories per day depending on the type of exercise you are doing. On the other hand, if you are exercising on a daily basis and are looking to lose weight then you should subtract an additional 300 calories from your daily intake. This will help you to not only lose weight, but also to maintain muscle mass in the process.

Specific exercise plans

Strength Protocol 1*:* In this plan, you normally fast through the evening, the night and the morning. After you are *twelve hours into your fast*, exercise for one hour.

There are four primary exercises that you do during this workout. They are weighted chin ups, bench press, squat, and deadlift. Don't over complicate things by adding other types of exercises.

Weighted chin ups – Start with pulldowns, chins and then weighted chins, depending on your relative strength. Start loading with five to ten pounds after you are able to do eight body weight repetitions. Stay between four and six reps. Chins are considered better than pull-ups. Close-grip chins are also beneficial. You can focus on weighted chins and close-grip chins if you want to build up your biceps.

Bench press – You bench press to build up your chest, shoulders and triceps. If you struggle with bench press as a lot of beginners do, you can do dumbbell presses or weighted dips as a substitute exercise. Barbell exercises such as bench press have the advantage of allowing you to progress with smaller weight jumps, though. You can also incorporate secondary shoulder movements such as overhead press or overhead dumbbell press, however these should be kept to a maximum of 3 working sets per workout.

Squats – The single best lower body muscle building exercise. In order to execute a proper squat, you should keep your trunk upright, your spine in a neutral position and your shoulders relaxed. You will also want to point your toes outward while setting your feet at hip width. From there, you will want to slowly lower your body down as you start the squat with the hips before following through with your knees. It is important to keep your core tight throughout this process, by taking a breath and holding it as you push your belly button backwards. This will help to protect your spine and create increased stability for your lower back.

It is also important to ensure the weight ends up being placed on your heels by driving your hips in behind you. While lowering yourself it is important to ensure your knees remain lined up with your big toe and that you do everything you can to ensure your knees don't buckle inward. Continue this motion until your hips are parallel to the floor before pushing up with your heels and returning to the starting position. Once there, you will want to exhale.

Squatting barefoot or in flat soled shoes (such as Converse sneakers) helps you maintain better form as regular running shoes have angled soles which can shift your weight forward.

Deadlift – Start by standing with your midfoot beneath the bar and stand so your hips are slightly more narrowed than when doing a squat. Point your toes so they are pointed slightly outward. Bend over without bending your legs to grab the bar. Grip it so your arms are about shoulder length apart. Your arms should be vertical when seen from the front. Drop into position through a knee bend and ensure you are low enough for your shins to touch the bar, taking special care to ensure the bar doesn't leave your midfoot. With a firm grip, straighten your back by raising your chest. Do this without changing position and ensuring the bar remains above your foot the entire time. Take a deep breath prior to standing up with the weight. The bar should maintain contact with your legs as you do so.

Return the weight to the floor by focusing on unlocking your knees and hips first. Lower the bar by moving your hips backward and keeping your legs straight. After the bar passes your knees, bend your legs even more. The bar should land on the ground directly over your midfoot

Note: With compound exercises like these, be sure to take appropriate rest between of three to five minutes between sets. When your strength improves, your muscles build. Either do a conditioning session or a strength session, but don't do both in the same session or else you will become only mediocre at both. Change parameters from week to week. Keep a training log and go for PRs on a regular basis.

Strength Protocol 2: Do three sets for ten reps for four of the following exercises:

Leg extensions: For this exercise, you are going to need to use a leg extension machine. As you exhale, you are going to want to flex your quadriceps and extend your leg to its maximum length. Once your leg is fully extended you are going to want to lower the weight back to its original position slowly so that you remain in control, inhaling as you do so. It is important that you do not go past a 90-degree angle. Repeat as needed.

Dumbbell lunges: Hold a dumbbell in each hand so your arms hang naturally at your sides. Stand upright, holding your torso erect, and step forward with your dominant leg about 2 feet while your other leg in its original spot. Lower your body down until the knee of your back leg touches the ground, moving slowly to maintain your balance. Return to a standing position and repeat with both legs.

Seated calf raises: This exercise requires a machine. Start by sitting on the machine with your towns on the lower platform with your heels from it. Place your thighs beneath the leer pad before placing your hands atop the pad to prevent slippage. Breath in as you slowly lower your heels by bending your ankles until your calves reach full extension. Raise your heels and extend your ankles as high as they will go before contracting your calves and releasing your breath. Hold this position for a few seconds and repeat as needed.

Seated rows: To do this exercise you need a low pulley row machine that comes equipped with a V bar. Sit down at the machine in such a way that your knees are bent slightly and are not locked. Grab hold of the V bar utilizing a neutral grip where the palms of your hands face one another. Fully extend your arms and pull back until your torso reaches a 90-degree angle from your legs. You will want to ensure that your back is lightly arched and your chest is sticking out. Keep your torso stationary and pull the handles towards your torso while at the same time keep your arms close to it until you come into contact with your abs, breathing out while you do so and contracting your back muscles. Hold for a moment and then return to the starting position.

Pull-ups: Grip the bar with your arms extended to about shoulder-width and your palms facing down. Bend your knees so that you are hanging with your feet off of the floor and your arms straight. Pull yourself up by drawing your elbows towards the floor while keeping them close as well. Continue pulling until your chin is above the bar. Lower yourself in a controlled manner back towards the ground. Take a breath and repeat.

One-arm dumbbell preacher curl: Hold a dumbbell in one hand at arm's length and place your arm on top of an incline bench. While breathing in, lower the dumbbell by extending your upper arm completely. While exhaling, make use of your bicep to return the dumbbell to shoulder height. To ensure a full rep, make sure to bring your small finger higher than your thumb. Squeeze for 1 second in this position and return the dumbbell slowly to the starting position. Switch arms between each repetition.

Barbell bench press-wide grip: On a flat bench, lie back in such a way that your feet are firm on the floor. Take a wide grip on the bar with your palms facing forwards with a grip that is slightly less than shoulder width. Lift the bar and hold it with your arms locked above your head so the bar is perpendicular to the floor. Lower the bar to your chest slowly while breathing in. Hold the bar in place for 1 second before exhaling and returning the bar to the starting position, contracting your chest muscles as you do so. Ensure that it takes twice as long to bring the bar to your chest as it does to return it to the starting position.

Pushups with feet elevated: Lie on the floor facing down and place your hands at slightly-greater than shoulder width. Place your toes on an elevated flat surface. The greater the height of the flat surface, the more resistance you will find in the exercise. Using just your arms, lower yourself downwards until your chest is almost touching the floor, inhaling while you do so. Flex your pectoral muscles and return your body to the starting position, exhaling while you do so. Pause for a moment and then repeat.

Front dumbbell raises: Pick up two dumbbells, one in each hand, and stand straight with the weights on your thighs at arm's length. They should be gripped so that your palms are facing your thighs. Keep your torso stationary while lifting one of the dumbbells in a forward motion using a slight bend of the elbow. Continue until your arm is slightly north of parallel to the ground, exhaling as you do so. Inhale as you lower the dumbbell back to the starting position before repeating with the dumbbell held in the other arm. For additional resistance you can attempt both arms at the same time.

Strength Protocol 3: Strength train for 30 minutes. Do two sets for five reptitions each of three of the following exercises:

Squats: See above.

Pull-ups: See above.

Elevated push-ups: See above.

Then follow up with 2 of these 3 exercises until your allotted time has expired.

Jump squat: Holding a pair of dumbbells in such a way that your palms face one another. Lower yourself into a squat position before launching yourself into the air with as much force as you can muster. Take care to land softly with your knees bent. Stand before returning to the starting position and repeat as needed.

Sprints: After a brief warmup, run 10, 200-meter intervals with of a goal of making each in less than 36 seconds. Rest for 30 seconds between intervals. Decrease resting time as you improve.

Frog jumps: With your hands behind your head, squat from a standing position so that your head is facing straight ahead and your torso is straight. Jump forward, focusing on distance instead of height. Absorb the impact with your legs as your feet come into contact with the ground. Repeat for 1 minute before resting for 15 seconds.

Chapter 8: Different Intermittent Fasting Daily Schedules

16/8

Number of fasting days – You diet for 7 days per week, partially fasting. Note: It is actually a full fast except for the BCAA protein shake in the morning when you exercise.

Meal schedule – You start this diet right after dinner and do a partial fast for 16 hours. For example, you may finish your dinner at 8pm, sleep for the night, skip breakfast (except for the three times that you get 10 grams of protein) and then eat lunch at noon.

Fasting day calories – Every day is a partial fasting day on this diet. There is no calorie counting to do on this diet, but you do measure out the 10 grams of protein that you get three times every morning.

5 days off/2 days on

Number of fasting days – You diet for one or two days per week.

Meal schedule – You completely stop eating for 24 hours on your fasting day(s). People commonly fast for fewer hours than 24 when they first start this diet.

You can start this diet by fasting only 15 hours for one day a week. Fast for 16 hours the next week. Add one more hour of fasting the next week and keep adding an hour every week until you can go without food for 24 hours for one day a week. Fast for 15 hours on a second, but non-consecutive, day of the week and work up to 24 hours of fasting on that second day.

Start your fasts after dinner. Skip breakfast and lunch the next day. Then break the fast with dinner the next day.

Fasting day calories – This is a full fast with no calories consumed at all on these days. Black coffee, water and unsweetened green tea are acceptable.

20/4

Number of fasting days – You diet for 7 days per week, partially fasting.

Meal schedule – You partially fast for 20 hours, starting after a late-night dinner. You nibble during the day and feast on all food groups late at night during a four-hour window.

Fasting day calories – You do not count calories on this diet.

Alternate Day Fasting

Number of fasting days – You diet for 3 non-consecutive days per week, partially fasting. People usually choose Monday, Wednesday, and Friday to fast while on this plan, leaving the two consecutive weekend days as normal eating days.

Meal schedule - There are no rules on this diet as far as the number of meals go or the time that you eat is concerned.

Fasting day calories - Consume 500 calories if you are a man and 400 calories if you are a woman on your partial fasting days.

The 5:2 Diet

Number of fasting days – You diet for 2 non-consecutive days per week, partially fasting. Pick any two days of the week and try to stick with those days every week.

Meal schedule – Divide your allotted calories between two meals on the days that you fast.

Fasting day calories – Consume 600 calories if you are a man and 500 calories if you are a woman on your partial fasting days.

Building A Successful Fasting Mindset

While each type of intermittent fasting is beneficial in its own way, they can all feel both complicated and difficult to stick with if you don't approach them with the proper mindset. The following suggestions will make the process much easier to manage.

Be true to yourself: Just because intermittent fasting has the possibility to offer you the type of healthy lifestyle you are looking for, this in no way means that it is going to be compatible with your personality, habits and schedule. While you will likely be able to make it through a handful of fasts without giving in to the temptation to break them early, while doing so it is important to consider how difficult it was for you to follow through on, what your general relationship with food is like and what your natural eating patterns are. It is also important to keep in mind that intermittent fasting is a lifestyle, not a diet you are going to stick with for a short period of time and then discard.

As such, it is important that you take the time to have a conversation with yourself and determine if the internal and external factors that affect you ever day are going to align in such a way that fasting regularly is a realistic proposition. Regardless of what you ultimately decide, it is important to make the decision relatively early on as changing your eating patterns too regularly can have negative consequences for your body.

When making this decision you are also going to need to take into account your overall level of discipline as well as your overall level of health. For example, if you feel as though you have a lot of weight to lose, starting with something less extreme than intermittent fasting might be a better choice until you are already moving in the right direction. Starting off with a diet plan that has such a high learning curve can be detrimental to your weight loss goals if you fail to live up to the strict regulations early on.

Failing in this fragile state could actually set you back in terms of overall progress and make it harder to continue pushing forward in the long run.

Be in touch with your body: While it is normal to experience negative side effects when your body is first adapting to new eating patterns, it is still important to take what your body is telling you into account to ensure you don't accidentally do more harm than good in the process. This is true during the first month of intermittent fasting when you are more likely to feel irritable, angry, weak, faint, lightheaded or shaky.

While it is likely that you will experience some of these symptoms to one degree or another, it is important to not push yourself too far, too fast and if any of them become too much and instead give your body a rest before continuing. Maintaining your overall health is a crucial part of successfully fasting intermittently in the long turn and pushing yourself to the verge of literally passing out from hunger is never a good idea, regardless of the circumstances.

Keep your expectations measurable: While the first month or two of your intermittent fasting plan will likely come with larger than average weight loss totals, you are going to need to keep in mind that they are going to taper off once your body gets used to the new eating pattern. Instead of trying to starve yourself in order to keep it up, it is important to instead become used to the fact that any diet should only result in between 1 and 2 pounds of healthy weight loss per week. Anything more than that is simply unhealthy.

Furthermore, you will want to keep in mind that any form of dieting is also going to come with weight loss plateaus where you likely won't lose anything for a week or two at a time. It is important to stay the course when this occurs as opposed to making radical changes to your diet based on a temporary loss of effectiveness. Failing to stay the course in this scenario is only going to lead to scenarios where your body shuts down all weight loss out of confusion for what exactly is going on. Slow and steady will win the race every time, stay the course and your weight loss will always get back on track eventually.

If your weight loss plateaus for 3 weeks or more, then a diet reset is the best solution for both your physical and mental health. During this period you should stick to your IF protocol and fast at the same time, but you can be more relaxed on your food choices during your eating periods. While this may seem counter-intuitive in the short-term, it has innumerable long term benefits. Diet resets should be taken at least twice a year for a 1 week period.

Don't make excuses: While it is important to not try intermittent fasting for the first time when your schedule is extremely busy, it is also important to not use minor reasons for not getting started keep popping up time and again. If this is the case then these reasons are more likely to be thinly-veiled excuses and the longer you abide by them the more difficult it will be to actually get started fasting.

Eventually, you are just going to need to tell yourself that enough is enough and get down to the business of doing your first intermittent fast. Remember, the only person who can motivate you to stick with it in the long run is you. This is why it is so important to not let yourself down and commit to finding the success that can be achieved by finally succeeding when it comes to the weight loss goals of your dreams.

Ensure your goals are realistic: Once you have managed to start using an intermittent fasting meal plan effectively, it is important that you don't expect too much from the plan too soon. Most importantly, 3,500 calories is a pound of fat but that type of loss doesn't take muscle building into account meaning that if you are exercising at the same time it is only logical that sometimes your weekly total is going to be less than it otherwise would be. This will happen despite the fact that you are feeling and looking better than you did before.

If you find yourself feeling discouraged when it comes to a presumed lack of results, you should take a moment and consider how long it took you to get to the point you are at now. With that amount of time in mind, you will then want to ask yourself why you would possibly expect to be able to reach your goals in less time than it took for you to gain the excess weight in the first place. Keeping a realistic perspective on the situation will make it much easier to follow through during the early days and thus, more effectively turn your new way of eating into a lifelong habit.

Take it slow: If you have never gone more than 12 hours without eating prior to your first day of intermittent fasting then you are most likely going to be better off starting at the 12-14 hour point and working your way up from there. Starting with a more extreme form of intermittent fasting is akin to going from 0 to 60 without going through the intervening gears required to get there without burning out. Remember, there is no time frame when it comes to intermittent fasting, simply stick with whatever works for you.

Conclusion

You have learned many things about intermittent fasting and how to use this technique to lose weight and to gain muscle. You have sample meal schedules that you can use to help to get you on the path to health and to a better self-image.

You may want to read this material one or two more times, and make some choices as to what your goals will be. Do you want to lose a lot of weight? Do you want a combination of weight loss while being able to retain your muscle mass?

Next, decide how you will go about reaching those goals. Schedule in the times of exercise, and determine the schedule you will use to eat and what food you will eat.

Then write out meal plans, and make a grocery list of the ingredients you will need to make the first week's planned meals. You may even re-use that grocery list and the ones you make out in the following weeks until you memorize the various recipes to meals you will want to eat repeatedly in the future.

Buy the food you will eat during your first week, and be sure to get rid of any junk food and extra carbohydrate food that is in your kitchen. Make your first meal according to the plan you worked out for yourself. Cook the next meal. Take it one meal and one day at a time until you have formulated healthy habits and your body starts to crave "real" food and exercise.

Finally, if you found this book useful, I would greatly appreciate it if you would review this book on Amazon.

Thank you for reading.

Keto Meal Prep

How to Save $100 and 4 Hours A Week by Batch Cooking

By

Jason Michaels

Introduction

Welcome and thank you for purchasing a copy of *Keto Meal Prep*.

The world we live in today is all about hustling to the next opportunity and bustling through the inevitable daily to-do list. While we are succeeding in our careers and family life, we are failing our health by fueling our bodies with fatty convenience store snacks, and fast food eats loaded with extra sugars and carbs.

Now is not the time to blame yourself but realize that you only have one body in this lifetime and you need to begin treating it like the beautiful temple of life it is! But how does someone who is constantly busy and on-the-go eat healthier? Well, I am glad you asked!

The chapters within this book hold two incredible sources of getting your health back on track into one jam-packed book of valuable information and recipes! Let me introduce you to the ketogenic diet, paired with the awesome convenience and power of meal prepping!

The following chapters will discuss what the ketogenic diet is and how it can help you get your life back on track and feeling your best! But the best part of this book will teach you the basics of meal prepping and how it can drastically change the way you fuel your body; with meal prep, there are no excuses when it comes to choosing healthier meal choices because you already did all the work yourself!

Thanks again for your interest in how meal prepping on the ketogenic diet can change your life! Every effort was made to ensure it is full of as much useful information as possible, please enjoy!

Jason Michaels

Chapter 1: Brief Overview of the Keto Diet

This is a high-fat diet that this is low in carbs and moderate in protein consumption. The ketogenic is based on the metabolic state that you aim to get your body into, known as *ketosis*.

When your body is successfully in a ketosis state, the liver produces ketones, which become your body's main source of energy. The core of the keto is based around the idea that the human body was created to run better as a fat burner rather than a burner of sugar and carbs for energy. The ketogenic diet reverses the way in which your body functions in a positive manner. This means that it has the power to totally change your perspective on healthy nutrition!

Fat Torch Versus Sugar Burner

When you consume items that are high in carbs, such as that daily morning donut, your body has to create insulin and glucose to break it down:

- *Insulin* is created to help process the glucose in the bloodstream by transporting it throughout the body.

- *Glucose* is a molecule that is easily converted by the body as an energy source.

When glucose is the body's primary source of energy, fats are not needed, which means they are stored, also known as that pesky excess weight you want to rid yourself of. When your body uses all its glucose, your brain signals you to reach for a snack, which is typically unhealthy such as chips or candy.

This is where the ketogenic diet has the power to reverse the effects of unhealthy eating by transforming your body into a fat burner instead of a sugar burner. When you lower your consumption of carbohydrates, your body then tries to find another energy source, which is when your body enters ketosis.

When your body reaches the state of ketosis, fat cells release any water that they had been storing and the fat cells can make an entrance into the bloodstream and go to the liver. This is essentially the goal of the keto diet. Despite popular belief, you cannot enter ketosis by starving your body, but rather by not consuming carbohydrates.

Keto Diet Benefits

- More effective weight loss
- Improved cholesterol levels
- Decrease in insulin levels
- Improved blood sugar levels
- Elimination of diabetes precursors
- Decrease in the development of diseases like Parkinson's and Alzheimer's
- Treatment for cancer and growth of tumors
- Treatment for reducing symptoms of epilepsy
- Healthier skin

Foods to Avoid

- *Sugary foods*: cake, soda, candy, fruit juice, ice cream, etc.

- *Grains and starches*: anything wheat and corn-based produce such as pasta, rice, and cereals

- *Fruit*: most fruits excluding berries

- *Beans and legumes*: peas, lentils, chickpeas, kidney beans, etc.

- *Root vegetables and tubers*: carrots, parsnips, potatoes, etc.

- *Condiments*

- *Unhealthy fats*: vegetable oils, mayonnaise, etc.

- *Alcohol*

- *Anything labeled "sugar-free," "diet," or "low-carb"*: these items contain sugar alcohols that can greatly affect the success of reaching ketosis

Food to Embrace

- *Meat*: red meat, chicken, steak, turkey, sausage, ham, bacon, etc.

- *Fish*: salmon, trout, tuna, and mackerel

- *Cream and butter*: Grass-fed is the best

- *Nuts and seeds*: chia seeds, almonds, pumpkin seeds, walnuts, flaxseeds, etc.

- *Healthy oils*: extra virgin olive, coconut, avocado, etc.

- *Herbs and spices*

- *Low-carb vegetables*: green veggies, tomatoes, avocados, onions, peppers, etc.

Chapter 2: Why You Should Be Meal Prepping

There are many people that aspire to live a healthier lifestyle but have no idea where to start or have no time to spare. Eating healthy is one thing, but following through with your health and fitness goals and staying consistent is challenging.

When you have your hands full navigating life, cooking all our own meals can feel impossible, and the temptations of hitting up a fast food joint seem like an easier option.

If you are ready to reach your fitness goals, stop spending extraordinary amounts of money on junk food, then your new best friend is meal prepping!

What is Meal Prepping?

Meal prepping is planning, preparing, and packaging snacks and meals for the upcoming week with the idea of portion control and clean eating in mind. No right or wrong way happens to meal prep, which makes it a great dieting alternative for busy bees to personalize to fit into their daily schedule.

The goal of meal prepping is to save substantial time slaving away in the kitchen while having access to healthier meal options throughout the week. You simply dedicate time to planning your meals and cooking their components. Besides that, you will become *amazed* at the difference meal prepping will make in your day to day life!

Reasons Why You Should Be Meal Prepping

Effective weight loss

When you plan your meals in advance, you will know what you are putting into your body. A meal prep routine lets you control how many calories you consume, which is essential for weight loss.

Saves money

Despite popular belief, eating healthy doesn't have to be pricey. Purchasing things in bulk and taking advantage of your freezer is the key. You know exactly what to buy instead of purchasing ingredients you don't need. Plus, with meals already made, you will save a _ton_ of money on fast food meals - up to $100 a week in some cases.

Shopping is simpler

Once you plan your week's meals, grocery shopping will be a breeze since you will have a list to stick to instead of wandering around the store.

Learn portion control

Meal prep teaches you how to balance what you put inside your body. When you pack your meals in containers, it keeps you from reaching for more food that you don't need. This is essential if you want to lose weight; meal prepping allows you to control the nutrients and calories you eat.

Less waste

Meal prepping lets you utilize all your ingredients for the week before they go bad! This is a much better alternative than trashing expensive produce before you have a chance to eat it.

Jason Michaels

Saves time

While you will need to set time aside to prepare your meals, you will end up saving time in the long run. Think about it; how much time do you spend with the fridge open? How much time do you waste making a decision of what to eat just to become a victim of tempting convenience foods? With meal prep, meals are prepared ahead of time, requiring you to remove from the fridge and nuke them in the microwave. Easy!

Investment in your health

When you can pick what you are going to stuff your face with ahead of time, you have ample time to make much healthier decisions. The benefits of eating cleaner are endless! Good nutrition is everything, especially if you are looking to fit into that bikini for the summer!

Strengthens willpower

Once you become accustomed to eating healthier, you will find that you no longer crave sugar and carbs. When you have a consistent routine of eating better, you will turn down unhealthy food choices much easier.

Reduces stress

Stress directly impacts your immune system, which can cause you to experience digestive issues, lack of quality sleep, and many more negative side effects. Coming home from work and having a meal ready to eat takes away that everyday stress!

Adds variety to your diet

Once you get the hang of meal prepping, you will feel more confident to try new recipes with new ingredients. Your taste buds will receive a variety of flavor daily.

Chapter 3: How to Avoid the 10 Most Common Meal Prep Mistakes

The way you approach meal prepping will make a world of difference when it comes to successfully implementing it into your everyday life. There are many tips out there regarding choosing recipes, shopping, and bringing it all together to create a week's worth of delicious eats.

However, you need to be aware of the things that could potentially go wrong and be knowledgeable of solutions to avoid meal prep pitfalls.

Mistake 1: Not giving yourself enough time to plan

Meal planning takes time and cannot happen in an hour. When you plan, shop, and prep as soon as you can, you are not giving yourself a sufficient amount of time to process everything, which can make it more of a stressful experience than it has to be.

- *Solution:* Allow yourself ample time to plan meals, especially as a beginner. Set aside 2 to 3 hours per week. Take advantage of the weekend to spread out planning, shopping, and prepping of meals. This will allow prepping to feel like a sustainable task that you can do for months to come. An easy way to do this at first is to make a meal calender for the upcoming week. This will help you plan efficiently and avoid wasting food.

Mistake 2: Not choosing the best recipes for your personal needs

To ensure that meal prepping works the best for you and your lifestyle, you need to understand the importance of what your body needs from the recipes you choose. If you pick a bunch of recipes that don't come close to the criteria, you will be hungry and unsatisfied.

- **Solution:** <u>Choose recipes</u> based on the meals you *need*. While this seems obvious, many people overlook this. Create a list of what you want recipes to do for you.

    o Need recipes to be 30 minutes or less?
    o Are you a vegetarian?

o What ingredients do you have that need to be used?

Mistake 3: Being unrealistic and too ambitious

Meal planning should be viewed as a marathon, not a sprint to the finish. You will feel super inspired at the start of your meal prep journey, but once you start to get into the depths of planning, you can become easily overwhelmed. You need to ensure that your prep schedule matches your regular schedule so that you can sustain it.

- **Solution:** Begin by creating defined goals and <u>assessing your daily routine</u> and schedule; this will help you to find what is realistic for *you*. Start small and start prepping two to three nights per week. This will give you the opportunity to figure out what works and what doesn't and allows you to tweak it to your liking.

Mistake 4: Not stocking the pantry

Experienced meal planners know how essential it is to always have meal basics on hand. If you fail to keep a good supply of staple items, you will miss all the benefits of meal planning and will likely become susceptible to temptation.

- **Solution:** Stock your pantry with all the basics that you can use time and time again in a variety of recipes:

    o Canned goods
    o White wine vinegar
    o Pepper, salt, and other spices
    o Canned tomatoes
    o Natural sweeteners (agave, maple, and honey)
    o Coconut milk
    o Olive oil
    o Stock
    o Etc.

Even on the days, you feel like you have nothing to consume, those basic components can help you create a yummy frittata, a delicious three-ingredient entre, or a one-pot wonder.

Mistake 5: Not searching for items that need to be used up

Before you head to the store, take an inventory of ingredients you already have in your kitchen and make use of leftover components you have. It's a simple step that helps you to prevent waste and saves you money.

- *Solution:* Before choosing recipes and making a grocery list, look in your cupboards, pantry, and fridge for food that needs to be used first. Turn those greens into a tasty side before going bad or thaw that pack of chicken to create a delicious main course.

Mistake 6: Not jotting down recipes

Meal prepping is all about being organized is you want to be successful. If you fail to save or write down recipes you have enjoyed, you will fall off track and become overwhelmed.

- *Solution:* Stay organized by keeping track of recipes that you have enjoyed and new ones you want to try out. It doesn't have to be fancy; could be a scrap piece of paper or on a whiteboard in your kitchen.

Mistake 7: Not taking inventory before shopping

Once you have picked your recipes for the week, you need to see what items you already have in your pantry. This is a closely tied mistake to not seeing the ingredients that need to be used before going bad.

- **Solution:** Before heading to the store, double check your recipe and the list of ingredients. Check your kitchen to ensure you don't have any of the components already so that you prevent overbuying.

Mistake 8: Skipping pre meal prep

Pre meal prepping is obviously an essential part of meal prep; this is small tasks like organizing ingredients and labelling containers. This gives your future self a giant hand. If you skip it, you are hurting yourself and leaves more work to do on the weekends.

- ***Solution:*** Set aside 30 minutes to an hour of prep each evening. This will make weekend meal prep a heck of a lot more efficient.

Mistake 9: Trying new recipes each day

I highly encourage you to try new recipes, but it's also important to go about eating a new variety of foods in a strategic way. When you fill up the whole week with brand new recipes, it can become very overwhelming and hard to sustain over a long period of time.

- ***Solution:*** Don't throw new recipes to the side but build your meal plan around recipes you know and then add 1 or 2 new recipes per week. This will help your taste buds from becoming bored and will also strengthen your recipe collection.

Mistake 10: Failing to have a backup plan

Even the most experienced meal preppers are bound to get stuck at work or have evenings where they are not feeling like consuming the dinner they planned out. Having a plan B is essential to stay the course.

- ***Solution:*** Have a good backup plan and have recipes in your back pocket that you know how to make. These will be very simple and can be made quickly, such as an omelet.

Jason Michaels

Chapter 4: Delicious Keto Recipes

The following sections withhold a wide array of delicious, easy-to-make keto meal prep recipes that you will certainly want to keep in that back pocket of yours! With these recipes, you will have fewer excuses when it comes to fueling your body in a way that makes you feel better both inside and out!

Breakfast Recipes

Greek Egg Bake

Protein: 15g Fat: 11g Net Carbs: 5g Calories: 175 Fiber: 9g

Ingredients:

- ¼ cup sun-dried tomatoes
- ½ cup feta cheese
- ½ tsp. oregano
- 1 cup chopped kale
- 12 eggs

Instructions:

1. Ensure your oven is preheated to 350 degrees.

2. With the foil, line a baking sheet and with the nonstick spray, spray well.

3. Whisk the eggs and then stir in the oregano, feta cheese, tomatoes, and kale.

4. In the sheet, pour the egg mixture. Then, bake the mixture for 25 minutes.

5. Let it cool and slice.

Can be served right away or kept in the fridge for 4 to 5 days.

Turmeric Scrambled Egg Meal Prep

Protein: 29g Fat: 18g Net Carbs: 6g Calories: 216 Fiber: 11g

Ingredients:

- ½ tsp. dried parsley

- 1 cup steamed broccoli

- 2 tbsps. coconut milk

- 2 tsp. dried turmeric

- 4 eggs

- 8 pre-cooked sausages

Instructions:

1. With the nonstick spray, grease a frying pan and then place it over medium heat setting.

2. Whisk the turmeric, parsley, milk, and eggs together with a pinch of the pepper and salt.

3. In the frying pan, slowly pour the mixture of eggs. Then cook well for 2 to 3 minutes, stirring the mixture constantly to break the eggs apart.

4. Flip the eggs and cook for another couple minutes till you reach the desired texture.

5. Add the eggs to two meal prep containers and add the veggies and sausage to the containers.

Can be refrigerated for up to 5 days.

Three-Ingredient Cauliflower Hash Browns

Protein: 7g Fat: 12g Net Carbs: 3.2g Calories: 164 Fiber: 2g

Ingredients:

- ¼ tsp. cayenne pepper

- 1 egg

- ¼ tsp. garlic powder

- ¾ cup shredded cheddar cheese

- ½ tsp. salt

- 1 head of cauliflower

- 1/8 tsp. pepper

Instructions:

1. Ensure your oven is preheated to 400 degrees. Grease a tray with the nonstick spray.

2. Grate the head of the cauliflower. For 3 minutes, place in the microwave and allow to cool. Ring out excess water with the cheesecloth or paper towels.

3. Place the cauliflower with the remaining ingredients and stir well to combine.

4. On a greased tray, form the mixture into square hash browns.

5. Bake for 15 to 20 minutes.

6. Let it cool for 10 minutes.

7. Serve it warm or place into the meal prep containers.

Can be refrigerated for 4 to 5 days.

Vegan Egg Muffins

Protein: 13g Fat: 9g Net Carbs: 4.1g Calories: 143 Fiber: 6g

Ingredients:

- ¼ cup coconut milk
- ½ thinly sliced sweet onion
- ½ tsp. dried oregano or 1 tsp. fresh oregano
- ¾ cup chopped red bell peppers
- ¾ tsp. sea salt
- 1 ½ cup fresh spinach
- 8-ounce pork breakfast sausage
- 1 tbsp. extra virgin olive oil

- 9 eggs

Instructions:

1. Ensure your oven is preheated to 350 degrees. Grease a muffin tin.
2. Sauté the ground sausage, breaking up as it cooks.
3. When halfway cooked, add a tablespoon of the olive oil, along with the oregano, pepper, and onions. Sauté the mixture till the onions turn into translucent.
4. Cover the pan after adding the spinach. Cook for 30 seconds and then toss the mixture. Spinach should be wilted. Take the pan off the heat.
5. Mix the eggs in a bowl with the milk, pepper, and salt, whisking till well beaten.
6. To the eggs, add the cooked sausage and veggie mixture and mix till well combined.
7. In a muffin tin, put the mixture evenly.
8. Bake for 18 to 20 minutes.

Refrigerate for up to 4 days and frozen for up to 2 months.

Turkey Chorizo Breakfast Sandwich

Protein: 29g Fat: 11g Net Carbs: 8g Calories: 203 Fiber: 5g

Ingredients:

Turkey Chorizo:

- ¼ tsp. cayenne pepper
- 1 tsp. coriander
- ¼ tsp. dried thyme
- ¼ tsp. cinnamon
- ½ tsp. dried oregano
- ¼ tsp. pepper
- ¼ tsp. onion powder
- 1 tbsp. cumin
- 1 tsp. fennel seeds
- 1 tbsp. paprika
- 1 tsp. sea salt
- 1/8 tsp. cloves, ground
- 1-pound turkey breast, lean ground
- 1 tsp. garlic powder

Breakfast Sandwich:

- ¼ avocado
- 1 cooked turkey chorizo patty
- 1 egg
- 1 whole wheat English muffin

Instructions:

1. *To make the chorizo:* In a bowl, add the turkey and spices. Mix them well with your clean hands. Create 16 even-sized portions and make them into ¼-inch patties.
2. Cook the chorizo patties in a greased skillet till the patties turn brown.
3. *To make a sandwich:* Spray a skillet and add the egg. Cook to your preference.
4. Toast your English muffin.
5. Serve the muffin topped with one chorizo patty, eggs, and avocado.

Freeze the remaining patties to enjoy throughout the week.

Banana Strawberry Baked Oatmeal

Jason Michaels

Protein: 14g Fat: 16g Net Carbs: 7g Calories: 154 Fiber: 11g

Ingredients:

- 2 eggs
- ¼ cup pure maple syrup
- ½ tsp. salt
- 1 ½ cup chopped strawberries + more to serve
- 1 tsp. cinnamon
- 2 tsp. vanilla extract
- 3 cups almond milk
- 3 mashed/ripe bananas
- 4 cups oats, old-fashioned
- 1 tsp. baking powder

Instructions:

1. Ensure your oven is preheated to 350 degrees. Grease a baking dish.
2. Whisk the salt, baking powder, cinnamon, vanilla, maple syrup, milk, eggs, and banana together well.
3. Mix in the oats. Gently fold in the strawberries.
4. In the prepared dish, pour the mixture. Then, bake the mixture for 35-40 minutes till the oatmeal sets.

5. Before serving, allow it to sit for 5 minutes. Then, serve the topping with more chopped strawberries.

Leftovers can be refrigerated for 3 days.
Simply reheat the oatmeal with a bit of the almond milk and top with desired fruit if you so choose.

Banana Muffins

Calories: 134 Protein: 11g Net Carbs: 9.8g Fiber: 9g Fat: 4g

Ingredients:

- ¼ tsp. salt
- 1 tsp. vanilla extract
- ½ tsp. baking soda
- ½ cup unsweetened applesauce
- 1 ½ cup ripe bananas
- 3 tbsps. olive oil
- 1 tsp. baking powder
- 1 egg
- 1 1/3 cup wheat flour, whole

Instructions:

1. Ensure your oven is preheated to 375 degrees. Grease a muffin tin well.
2. Light beat the egg and then add the bananas, mashing well. Stir the remaining components, minus the flour.
3. Then add the flour, stirring gently till well combined. DON'T OVERMIX.
4. In the muffin tin, pour the batter.
5. Then, bake the batter for 22 minutes.

Muffins can either be refrigerated for 7 days or frozen for 3 months.

Vanilla Cinnamon Protein Bites

Protein: 2g Fat: 9g Net Carbs: 4.2g Calories: 112 Fiber: 3g

Ingredients:

- ¼ - 1/3 cup nut butter of choice (the creamier, the better!)
- ¼ - 1/3 cup pure maple syrup
- ¼ cup vanilla protein powder
- ½ cup almond meal

- ½ - 1 tsp. vanilla extract
- ¾ cup quick oats
- 1 tbsp. cinnamon

Instructions:

1. Grind the oats in your food processor and pour them into a mixing bowl. Add the nut butter, cinnamon, protein powder, and almond meal to the bowl, stirring well.
2. Pour in the vanilla and syrup, combining well with your clean hands.
3. With the parchment paper, like a cookie sheet, roll the mixture making 1 ½-inch balls and place on the lined sheet.
4. Freeze for 20 to 30 minutes and then place in a Ziploc baggie.
5. Dust the balls with the vanilla protein and cinnamon.

Can be refrigerated for 3 weeks or frozen for up to 6 months.

Low-Carb Breakfast Pizza

Jason Michaels

Protein: 19g Fat: 16g Net Carbs: 7.2g Calories: 307 Fiber: 5g

Ingredients:

- ¼ tsp. pepper
- ½ cup heavy cream
- ½ tsp. salt
- 1 cup shredded cheese of choice
- 12 eggs
- 2 cups sliced peppers
- 8 ounces of sausage

Instructions:

1. Ensure your oven is preheated to 350 degrees.
2. Microwave the peppers for 3 minutes.
3. In a cast iron skillet, brown the sausage. Set to the side.
4. Mix the pepper, salt, cream, and eggs together and place in the skillet.
5. Cook for 5 minutes till the sides begin to become firm.
6. Place the skillet in the oven and back for 15 minutes. Then, remove the skillet from the oven.

7. To the skillet, add the cheese, peppers, and sausage and then for 3 minutes, place it under the broiler.
8. Allow to sit for 5 minutes to cool. Devour right away or split between the meal prep containers.

Can be refrigerated for 5 days or frozen for 60 days.

Blueberry Pancake Bites

Protein: 6g Fat: 13g Net Carbs: 7.5g Calories: 188 Fiber: 4g

Ingredients:

- ½ cup frozen blueberries
- 1/3 – ½ cup water
- ½ tsp. cinnamon
- 1 tsp. baking powder
- ¼ cup melted ghee
- ½ tsp. salt
- ½ cup coconut flour
- ½ tsp. vanilla extract
- 4 eggs

Instructions:

1. Ensure your oven is preheated to 325 degrees. With the butter and coconut oil spray, grease a muffin tin.
2. Mix the vanilla, sweetener, and eggs together until smooth.
3. Stir in the cinnamon, salt, baking powder, melted ghee, and coconut flour, blending till smooth.
4. To the batter, add 1/3 cup of the water and blend once more. The batter should be thick.
5. Among the muffin tin cups, divide the batter and then add a few blueberries to each muffin.
6. For 20 to 25 minutes, bake until set.
7. Allow to cool.

Can be kept in a slightly cold place in an airtight container for 8-10 days. Can be frozen for 60-80 days.

Lunch Recipes

Shredded Chicken for Meal Prep

Calories: 115 Sugar: 0g Carbs: 0g Total Fat: 4g Protein: 19g

Ingredients:

- ½ tsp. black peppercorns
- 2 bay leaves
- 2 halved cloves of garlic
- 32 ounces of chicken broth (preferably reduced-sodium)
- 4 ½ - 5 pounds skinned chicken thighs
- 4 parsley stems
- 4 thyme sprigs

Instructions:

1. Put the chicken in your slow cooker.
2. In a double-wrapped cheesecloth, place the peppercorns, garlic, bay leaves, parsley stems, and thyme sprigs. Tie off the cheesecloth and add the filled bouquet to the slow cooker.
3. Pour the broth into your slow cooker over the chicken and wrapped herbs.
4. Cover them and set to cook on low heat setting for 7 to 8 hours.
5. Discard the bouquet.
6. Place the chicken in a bowl and leave the cooking liquids in the cooker.
7. Once some of the chicken has cooled, take out the bones from the meat. Use two forks to shred the

chicken, adding reserved cooking liquids while
shredding to keep the meat moist.

8. Strain the remaining liquids and use for the future
stock if desired.

*Can be used in a large variety of meal prep recipes! To
make ahead, place 2 cups of stock and chicken in separate
containers.*

Can be frozen for 3 months and refrigerated for 3 days.

Easy Sheet Pan Roasted Vegetables

*Calories: 97 Protein: 2g Carbs: 11g Total Fat: 6g Sugar:
4g*

Ingredients:

- 1 tbsp. balsamic vinegar
- ¼ tsp. pepper
- 1 chopped red onion
- 1 tsp. coarse salt
- 2 chopped red bell peppers
- 2 tsp. Italian seasoning
- 3 tbsps. olive oil, extra virgin

- 3 cups cubed butternut squash
- 4 cups broccoli florets

Instructions:

1. Ensure your oven is preheated to 425 degrees.
2. Toss the cubed squash in a tablespoon of the oil and spread out onto a baking tray. Roast for 10 minutes.
3. Toss the pepper, salt, Italian seasoning, onion, bell peppers, and broccoli till coated well.
4. Add the roasted squash to the veggies. Toss well to incorporate. Spread the veggie mixture over two baking trays.
5. Roast for 17 to 20 minutes, making sure to stir around 1-2 times throughout the cooking process. Vegetables should be tender and browned in areas.
6. Drizzle with the vinegar before eating.

Can be refrigerated for up to 7 days.

Mango Coconut Chicken Bowls

Calories: 482 Sugar: 0g Carbs: 72g Total Fat: 8g Protein: 34g

Ingredients:

- ¼ cup sweetened shredded coconut
- 1 sliced avocado
- 2 cups cooked brown rice
- 4 chicken breasts (sliced lengthwise in half)

Mango marinade:

- 1 tsp. salt
- 2 tbsps. lime juice
- 1 tbsp. Sriracha
- 2 minced garlic cloves
- 1 tbsp. honey
- 2 tbsps. olive oil
- 1 mango

Corn salsa:

- ¼ cup cilantro
- 1 can drained black beans
- ½ diced red pepper
- ¾ tsp. salt
- 1 ½ cup corn
- 1 diced red onion
- 1 tbsp. lime juice

Instructions:

1. Ensure your oven is preheated to 425 degrees.
2. Cook the rice as per the package instructions.
3. In a blender, mix all of the mango marinade ingredients together till combined.
4. Marinate the chicken in half of the mango mixture for 10 minutes.
5. Mix together the corn salsa ingredients.
6. On your baking tray, place the chicken and bake for 15-20 minutes till golden in color.
7. Slice the chicken and place into bowls, along with additional mango sauce, corn salsa, topped with the shredded coconut and cilantro. Place the avocado on top.

Can be chilled in your fridge up to 5 days.

Chicken Tikka Masala Prep Bowls

Calories: 215 Sugar: 2g Carbs: 17g Total Fat: 9g Protein: 21g

Ingredients:

Jason Michaels

- 1 ½ pounds chicken breasts (cut into 1-inch pieces; boneless, skinless)
- 1 cup brown rice
- 1 diced onion
- ¼ cup cilantro
- 1 tbsp. lemon juice
- 1 tbsp. ginger, grated
- 1/3 cup heavy cream
- 2 tbsps. tomato paste
- 1 cup chicken stock, reduced-sodium
- 2 tbsps. unsalted butter
- 2 tsp. garam masala
- 28-ounce can diced tomatoes
- 2 tsp. chili powder
- 3 minced garlic cloves
- 2 tsp. turmeric

Instructions:

1. Cook the rice in 2 cups of water following the package directions.
2. In a skillet, melt the butter. With the pepper and salt, season the chicken. Then, with the onion, add

the chicken to the skillet, cooking for 4 to 5 minutes till golden.

3. Stir in the turmeric, chili powder, garam masala, ginger, and tomato paste, cooking for 1 to 2 minutes as you combine.

4. Pour the chicken stock and tomatoes in. Bring the mixture to a boil.

5. Decrease heat. Then, for 10 minutes, let it simmer, stirring on occasion.

6. Mix in the lemon juice and cream, heating through 1 minute.

7. Spoon the rice and chicken into the meal prep bowls and garnish with the cilantro.

Refrigerated for up to 7 days or frozen for 1 month.

Spinach, Tomato, and Bacon Muffin Tin Quiche

Calories: 96 Carbs: 2g Sugar: 0g Protein: 13g Total Fat: 9g

Ingredients:

- ¼ cup tomatoes, diced
- ½ cup low-fat milk
- ½ tsp. pepper

- ½ cup chopped green onions
- ½ tsp. salt
- 1 ½ cup red-skinned potatoes, diced
- 2-ounces shredded cheese of choice
- 1 ½ cup chopped spinach
- 2 tbsps. extra virgin olive oil
- 3 strips of cooked/chopped bacon
- 8 eggs

Instructions:

1. Ensure your oven is preheated to 325 degrees. Liberally grease a muffin tin.
2. Set over medium heat, warm oil in a pan. To the pan, add some salt and potatoes, stirring for 5 minutes till the potatoes are just cooked. Take it off the heat. Allow to sit and cool for 5 minutes.
3. Whisk the pepper, salt, milk, cheese, and eggs together.
4. Fold in the cooked potatoes, tomatoes, green onion, and spinach to the egg mixture.
5. Pour the egg and veggie mixture evenly in your muffin tin.
6. Bake for 25 minutes till firm to the touch.
7. For 5 minutes, allow to sit.

Can be refrigerated for 3 days and frozen up to a month.

To reheat, remove the plastic wrapper, put a dampened paper towel around it, and then heat in the microwave for 30 to 60 seconds. Enjoy!

Taco Scramble

Calories: 450 Carbs: 24g Sugar: 3g Total Fat: 19g Protein: 46g

Ingredients:

- ¼ cup chopped scallions
- ¼ cup water
- ¼ tsp. adobo seasoning salt
- ½ cup Mexican shredded cheese
- ½ minced onion
- 1 pound lean ground turkey
- 2 tbsps. homemade taco seasoning (Tastier and better for you than the store-bought!)
- 2 tbsps. minced bell pepper
- 4-ounce can tomato sauce
- 8 beaten eggs

Potatoes:

- ½ tsp. garlic powder
- 1 pound red potatoes, quartered
- ¾ tsp. salt
- 4 tsp. olive oil

Homemade taco seasoning:

- 1 tsp. chili powder
- ½ tsp. oregano
- 1 tsp. paprika
- 1 tsp. cumin
- 1 tsp. garlic powder
- 1 tsp. salt

Instructions:

1. Beat the eggs, add the seasoning salt, and fold in the cheese.
2. Ensure your oven is preheated to 425 degrees. Grease a casserole dish.
3. Add the oil, salt, garlic powder, and 1-2 pinches of the pepper to the potatoes. Bake the potatoes for 45

minutes till tender, making sure to stir every 15 minutes.

4. Brown the turkey. Then add the water, tomato sauce, bell pepper, and onion. Stir, simmering for 20 minutes

5. Spray a separate skillet liberally using the cooking spray and add the eggs and ¼ teaspoon of the salt. Scramble for 2 to 3 minutes.

6. When serving, put ¾ cup of the turkey and 2/3 cup of the eggs into a meal prep container or serving bowl. Divide the potatoes among each serving with 1 tablespoon of the cheese and scallions.

Chicken Sausage and Peppers

Calories: 249 Protein: 18g Carbs: 20g Total Fat: 11g Sugar: 11g

Ingredients:

- 1 sweet onion (cut into wedges)
- 2 cups grape tomatoes
- 1 tbsp. oregano
- 1 tbsp. vinegar, balsamic

- 12-ounce package of Italian-flavored cooked chicken sausage
- 1 tbsp. olive oil
- 4 sweet peppers, color of choice (chop into 1-inch pieces)

Instructions:

1. Ensure your oven is preheated to 425 degrees. Liberally grease a baking pan.
2. In the prepared pan, add the tomatoes, onion, and peppers. Drizzle with the vinegar and olive oil and toss. Roast for 30 minutes.
3. Move the roasted veggies to one side of the tray and put the sausage in an empty portion. Roast for another 10 to 15 minutes till the sausage is heated through.
4. Sprinkle with the oregano.

Can be refrigerated for 7 days and frozen for 15 days.

Southwestern Chicken Burrito Bowls

Calories: 301 Sugar: 3g Carbs: 10g Total Fat: 14g Protein: 21g

Ingredients:

- ¼ tsp. cayenne
- ¼ tsp. pepper
- 1 ½ cup canned black beans
- ½ tsp. cumin
- ¾ cup canned corn
- 1 cup grape tomatoes
- 1 cup cooked rice
- 1 tsp. paprika
- 2 cups kale
- 3 cups shredded chicken

Instructions:

1. Prepare the rice according to the package instructions. Mix the pepper, cayenne, cumin, and paprika in with the rice when there are around 5 minutes left to cook the rice.
2. Layer your meal prep containers with the shredded chicken, rice, beans, corn, kale, and tomatoes.
3. Top with the dressing and enjoy it right away or store in the fridge for later enjoyment.

Can be refrigerated for 7-10 days.

Jason Michaels

Skinny Joes With Tangy Slaw

Calories: 381 Protein: 29g Carbs: 23g Total Fat: 14g Sugar: 4g

Ingredients:

- 1 cup chopped tomatoes
- ½ cup rolled oats
- 1 cup water
- 1 red onion, chop
- 1 green or red bell pepper, chop
- 1 ½ tsp. salt
- 1 grated carrot
- 1 tbsp. Worcestershire sauce
- 1-pound ground beef, lean
- 2 tsp. garlic powder
- 1 tbsp. olive oil
- 4 tbsps. apple cider vinegar
- 4 tbsps. tomato paste

Tangy Slaw:

- ½ chopped red onion

- ½ head cabbage
- 1 tbsp. honey
- 1 tbsp. mustard, Dijon
- 2 grated carrots
- 2 tbsps. apple cider vinegar

Instructions:

1. Press SAUTÉ. Pour the oil into an instant pot and allow to heat for a bit. Add the beef and cook till browned.
2. Push the beef to the side in the pot and add the garlic powder, salt, carrots, peppers, and onions, sautéing for 5 minutes till softened. Then pour in the water, tomato paste, chopped tomatoes, vinegar, and Worcestershire sauce. Mix well to incorporate.
3. When the mixture heats to boiling, toss in the oats. DO NOT STIR.
4. Close the lid. Press HIGH PRESSURE. For 10 minutes, cook the mixture.
5. Perform the natural release. Let it sit for a few minutes covered to allow to thicken.

1. *To make the slaw*, combine the honey, vinegar, and mustard.

2. Add the onions, carrots, and cabbage, tossing with the honey mixture.

Sloppy joe meat can be frozen for up to 3 months and refrigerated for 10 days.

Tangy slaw can be refrigerated for up to 4 days.

Mason Jar Recipes

Asian Chicken Mason Jar Salad

Calories: 524 Sugar: 15g Carbs: 39g Total Fat: 33g Protein: 28g

Ingredients:

- 1 1/3 cup halved snap peas
- 1 cup grated carrots
- 1 cup whole cashews, unsalted
- 1 julienned red pepper
- 2 cups baby spinach, sliced
- 2 cups napa cabbage, sliced
- 1 1/3 cup sliced cucumber
- 2 cups shredded rotisserie chicken

- 2 tbsps. green onions, sliced

Sesame dressing:

- 1 minced garlic clove
- 2 tbsps. rice vinegar
- 1 tbsp. minced ginger
- 1 tbsp. honey
- 1 tsp. sriracha sauce
- 1 tsp. sesame seeds
- 2 tbsps. cilantro
- 1 tbsp. olive oil
- 2 ½ tbsps. sesame oil , toasted
- 3 tbsps. low-sodium soy sauce
- *4 64-ounce mason jars*

Instructions:

1. Whisk the sesame seeds, honey, cilantro, garlic, ginger, sriracha, olive oil, toasted sesame oil, vinegar, and soy sauce together.
2. Toss the spinach and napa cabbage together.
3. Assemble the jars by adding 3 tablespoons of the dressing, 1/3 cup of the snap peas, ¼ cup of the chicken, ¼ cup of the cashews, and a sprinkle of the

green onion. Serve it now or place in the fridge. *Salads last 3 to 4 days in the fridge.*

Yogurt and Granola Parfait

Calories: 98 Sugar: 4g Carbs: 2g Total Fat: 4g Protein: 5g

Ingredients:

- 2 cups granola
- 2 cups Greek yogurt (any flavor)
- 4 cups berries

Instructions:

- Layer ½ cup of the granola, ½ cup of the yogurt, and 1 cup of the berries into the jar, continuously layering till you are out of ingredients.

Can be refrigerated for 3 to 4 days.

Zucchini Lasagna

Calories: 114 Sugar: 4g Carbs: 3g Total Fat: 9g Protein: 8g

Ingredients:

- ¼ cup minced parsley
- ½ cup diced onion
- ½ pound lean ground turkey
- ½ tbsp. Italian seasoning
- ½ tbsp. minced garlic
- ½ tsp. oregano
- 1 cup part-skim mozzarella cheese
- 1 egg yolk
- 2 tsp. salt
- 1 tbsp. olive oil
- 2 zucchinis
- 6 tbsps. canned tomato sauce
- 4 tsp. parmesan cheese
- 6 tbsps. crushed tomatoes
- 8 ounces low-fat ricotta cheese

Instructions:

1. Ensure your oven is preheated to 350 degrees.
2. Slice the zucchinis 1/8-inch thick and sprinkle with 1 ½ teaspoon of the salt.

3. Bake for 15-25 minutes till the water is released from edges.
4. Lay the zucchini out on paper towels. Reduce the oven temperature to 325 degrees.
5. In a pan, warm the olive oil. Then pour turkey, garlic, and onion, cooking the meat till cooked through. Season with the seasonings. Set it aside.
6. Mix the crushed tomatoes and tomato sauce together. With the salt and pepper, season.
7. Mix the pepper, salt, egg, and ricotta together as well.
8. Layer half of the sauce between four jars. Then layer the turkey, zucchini noodles, and other ingredients. Parsley and mozzarella should go on top. Seal the jars well.

Can be refrigerated for 3 days.

Berry and Nuts Salad

Calories: 92 Sugar: 3g Carbs: 0.5g Total Fat: 7g Protein: 10g

Ingredients:

*   ¼ cup chopped almonds

- ½ cup blackberries
- ½ cup blueberries
- ½ cup strawberries

Zesty Dressing:

- ¼ cup orange juice
- 1 tbsp. honey
- Juice and zest of a lemon
- 2 tbsps. olive oil

Instructions:

1. Whisk the dressing components together till blended.
2. In the mason jar, pour in 2-3 tablespoons of the dressing into the bottom. Then layer the berries, putting the almonds on the top.

Refrigerate for 3 days.

Asian Noodle Salad

Calories: 119 Sugar: 4g Carbs: 1g Total Fat: 5g Protein: 8g

Ingredients:

- ½ cup crunchy rice noodles
- 1 cup cooked/shelled edamame
- 4 green onions, sliced
- 2 carrots, peeled/shredded
- 4 ounces soba noodles

Spicy Peanut Dressing:

- ¼ cup olive oil, extra-virgin
- 4 tsp. vinegar, rice
- 2 tbsps. peanut butter
- 4 tsp. soy sauce
- 4 tsp. sambal

Instructions:

1. Whisk together all dressing components.
2. Pour the dressing into the bottom of the jar. Then layer the noodles, edamame, carrots, green onion, and noodles on top.

Refrigerate up to 4 days.

Mediterranean Salad

Calories: 201 Sugar: 2g Carbs: 2g Total Fat: 4g Protein: 13g

Ingredients:

- 1 cup whole-grain couscous, cooked
- 1 tbsp. olive oil
- 2 ounces crumbles feta cheese
- 4-5 slices artichoke hearts, marinated in olive oil
- 6-10 cherry tomatoes
- Juice of ½ a lemon
- Sea salt
- Sprinkle of dried basil, oregano, and parsley

Instructions:

1. Mix all liquid ingredients together to create a type of the dressing.
2. Pour the dressing into the bottom of the jar. Then add other ingredients to the jar as you see fit.

Refrigerate for up to 3 days.

Feta and Shrimp Cobb Salad

Calories: 192 Sugar: 5g Carbs: 2g Total Fat: 8g Protein: 11g

Ingredients:

- 1 chopped hard-boiled egg
- 1-2 handfuls baby spinach and romaine lettuce
- 1 tbsp. chopped red onion
- 2 chopped slices bacon
- 2 tbsps. avocado
- 2 tbsps. chopped cucumber
- 2 tbsps. crumbled feta cheese
- 6-8 boiled shrimps
- 8 grape tomatoes
- Vinaigrette of choice

Instructions:

1. Pour the vinaigrette into the bottom of the jar.
2. Then layer the veggies, shrimp, bacon, and cheese on top.

Refrigerate for up to 4 days.

BLT Salad

Calories: 205 Sugar: 6g Carbs: 6g Total Fat: 18g Protein: 17g

Ingredients:

- 14 croutons
- 2 cups iceberg lettuce
- 2 cups romaine lettuce
- 2 chopped scallions
- 2 chopped tomatoes
- 4 crumbled slices bacon

Instructions:

1. Whisk all dressing components together.
2. Pour the dressing into the bottom of the jar.
3. Layer the veggies, then the croutons and bacon on top and seal.

Refrigerate for 3 days.

Jason Michaels

Rainbow Salad

Calories: 109 Sugar: 0g Carbs: 1g Total Fat: 9g Protein: 15g

Ingredients:

- ½ cup raw sunflower seeds
- 1 cup sliced carrots
- 1 cup cucumber, chop
- 1 bell pepper, yellow, chop
- 1 bell pepper, red, chop
- 2 cups chopped red cabbage
- 8 cups assorted salad greens

Balsamic Dressing:

- ¼ cup chopped parsley
- ½ cup white balsamic vinegar
- 2 minced cloves garlic
- Pepper and salt
- 2 tbsps. olive oil

Instructions:

1. Whisk all of the dressing components together.

2. Drain the chickpeas.
3. Pour the dressing into the bottom of the jar. Then layer the veggies and sunflower seeds on top. Seal well.

Can be refrigerated for up to 5 days.

Spinach, Tomato, Mozzarella Salad

Calories: 184 Sugar: 3g Carbs: 3g Total Fat: 12g Protein: 11g

Ingredients:

- 10 cups baby spinach
- 10 ounces fresh mozzarella
- 1-quart grape tomatoes
- 10 tbsps. balsamic vinegar dressing

Instructions:

- Pour the dressing in the bottom of the jar.
- Load the jar with the veggies and then the cheese. Seal well.

Jason Michaels

Can be refrigerated for up to 3 days.

Dinner Recipes

Chipotle Turkey and Sweet Potato Chili

*Calories: 423 Carbs: 39g Total Fat: 18g Sugar: 6g
Protein: 28g*

Ingredients:

- ¼ - ½ tsp. ground chipotle powder
- 1 cup diced onion
- 1 tsp. oregano, dried
- 1 sweet potato
- 1 tbsp. oil, coconut
- 1 tsp. cumin
- 1-pound ground turkey
- 2 cups chicken broth
- 2 tsp. chili powder
- 28-ounces fire-roasted tomatoes
- 3 minced garlic cloves
- Pepper and salt

Instructions:

1. Warm up the coconut oil over intermediate-extreme warmth.

2. Once the oil begins to simmer, place the turkey in a pan. Cook for 5 minutes, breaking up as it cooks.

3. Toss in the garlic and onions, cooking for 8-10 minutes till the onions turn into translucent.

4. Turn the warmth up to high. Pour in the broth, sweet potato, and tomatoes, along with the seasonings. Bring the mixture up to a boiling point.

5. Turn down the heat to a medium setting and let simmer for 10-15 minutes uncovered. The longer you allow to simmer, the bigger the flavor.

Refrigerate for 7 days and freeze for up to 6 months.

Avocado Bacon Garlic Burger

Calories: 189 Sugar: 1g Carbs: 13g Total Fat: 22g Protein: 27g

Ingredients:

- ½ tsp. pepper
- 1 cup chopped basil
- 1 tsp. salt
- 1-pound grass-fed lean ground beef

Jason Michaels

- 2 eggs
- 3 minced cloves garlic

Toppings:

- 1 avocado
- 16 pieces of bacon, cooked
- 4 slices red onion

Instructions:

1. Mix all hamburger components till well incorporated.
2. Divide the meat into four patties.
3. In a pan, warm up the olive oil.
4. Then, place the patties, grilling for 4 minutes per side.
5. Make the burgers with the avocado as the bun and other desired toppings.

Chutney Cilantro Meatballs

Calories: 375 Sugar: 3g Carbs: 23g Total Fat: 29g Protein: 35g

Ingredients:

Sauce:

- ½ cup water
- 1 chopped yellow onion
- 2 tbsps. avocado oil
- 28-ounce can crushed tomatoes

Meatballs:

- ½ cup quick-cooking brown rice
- 1 tsp. salt
- 1 tsp. ras el hanout spice blend
- 1 pound ground turkey

Chutney:

- ¼ tsp. cayenne pepper
- 1 bunch cilantro
- 1 green onion
- ¼ tsp. pepper
- 1 tsp. sesame oil, toasted
- 1 tbsp. lemon juice
- ½ tsp. salt

Jason Michaels

Instructions:

1. To create the sauce, push SAUTÉ and warm up the oil. Sauté the onion for 10 minutes. Then add the water and tomatoes, mixing well as you heat to simmer.
2. To create the meatballs, mix the salt, ra el hanout, rice, and turkey together. Form the mixture into 12 meatballs.
3. Put the meatballs in an even layer in the simmering sauce, spooning a bit of the sauce over the meatballs.
4. Place the lid on, using the PRESSURE RELEASE to seal. Press CANCEL and select POULTRY for 15 minutes.
5. While the meatballs cook, prepare the chutney by combining all chutney ingredients together, grinding them into a paste with the mortar and pestle.
6. Perform the quick release on the meatballs. Serve in the sauce and top with the chutney.

Instant Pot Lamb Shanks

Calories: 338 Sugar: 6g Carbs: 19g Total Fat: 37g
Protein: 42g

Ingredients:

- ¼ cup minced Italian parsley
- 1 cup bone broth
- 1 chopped onion
- 1 tbsp. balsamic vinegar
- 1 tsp. fish sauce, red boat
- 1 pound ripe Roma tomatoes
- 1 tbsp. tomato paste
- 2 chopped celery stalks
- 2 tbsps. ghee
- 3 pounds lamb shanks
- 2 chopped carrots
- 3 smashed/peeled garlic cloves
- Pepper and salt

Instructions:

1. Season with the shanks with the pepper and salt.
2. Press SAUTÉ on the instant pot, melt a tablespoon of the ghee. Place the shanks into the pot and sear on all sides for 8-10 minutes.

3. As the lamb browns, chop up the veggies. Take out the lamb from the pot.

4. Lower the heat and add the remaining ghee. To the pot, add the onion, celery, and carrots, seasoning with the pepper and salt.

5. Add the garlic cloves and tomato paste, stirring for at least 60 seconds.

6. Place the shanks back into the pot along with the tomatoes.

7. Pour the balsamic vinegar, fish sauce, and bone broth into the pot.

8. Lock the lid. Press MANUAL and set to cook for 50 minutes. Perform the natural release.

9. Remove the shanks to the plate and top with the sauce.

Cranberry Spice Pot Roast

Calories: 312 Carbs: 13g Total Fat: 29g Sugar: 16g Protein: 54g

Ingredients:

- ¼ cup honey
- ½ cup water
- ½ cup white wine

- 1 cup frozen whole cranberries
- 1 tsp. horseradish powder
- 2 cups bone broth
- 2 peeled garlic cloves
- 2 tbsps. olive oil
- 3 to 4 pounds of beef arm roast
- 3-inch cinnamon stick
- 6 whole cloves

Instructions:

1. Dry the meat with the paper towels. Season liberally with the pepper and salt.
2. Press SAUTÉ on the instant pot. Heat up the oil and place the roast in, browning for 8-10 minutes on all sides. Remove and put to the side.
3. Pour the wine into the instant pot. Using a wooden spoon, from the bottom, scrape the bits. Cook for 4-5 minutes to deglaze.
4. Add the cloves, garlic, cinnamon stick, horseradish powder, honey, water, and cranberries to pot. Cook for 4-5 minutes till the cranberries start to burst open.
5. Place the meat back into the pot. Pour in just enough bone broth to cover the meat.

6. Lock the lid. Press HIGH PRESSURE to cook for 75 minutes.

7. Perform the natural release of the pressure for 15 minutes and then quick release the rest.

8. Place the meat on the serving platter and top with the cranberry sauce.

Garlic Pork and Kale

Calories: 437 Sugar: 11g Carbs: 20g Total Fat: 31g Protein: 49g

Ingredients:

- 1 tsp. minced rosemary
- 1 tbsp. red wine vinegar
- 20-25 whole garlic cloves
- 2 sprigs of thyme
- 1 chopped yellow onion
- 2 tbsps. olive oil
- 2 ½ pound pork shoulder (boneless; cut into 1 ½-inch chunks)
- 2/3 cup red wine, dry
- 2/3 cup chicken broth

Instructions:

1. Season the pork liberally with the pepper and salt.
2. Press SAUTÉ on the instant pot and heat up the olive oil. Working in batches, sear the pork till browned. Remove with the slotted spoon. Discard the fat from the instant pot.
3. Add the thyme and onion to the instant pot, sautéing for 5 minutes. Then add the rosemary and garlic, cooking for 60 seconds.
4. Using a wooden spoon, pour wine in to deglaze the bits from the bottom of the pot.
5. Pour in the broth and add the pork back in. Combine.
6. Lock the lid. Press MANUAL to cook for around 40 minutes. Perform the quick release.
7. Stir in the kale. Press HIGH PRESSURE to cook for another 10 minutes. Perform another quick release.
8. Kale and pork should be nice and tender.

Can freeze up to 3 months.

Lemon Pepper Salmon

Jason Michaels

Calories: 174 Sugar: 1g Carbs: 29g Total Fat: 11g Sodium: 118mg Protein: 36g

Ingredients:

- ¼ tsp. salt
- ½ thinly sliced lemon
- ½ tsp. pepper
- ¾ cup water
- 1 julienned carrot
- 1 julienned red bell pepper
- 1-pound salmon filet
- 1 julienned zucchini
- 3 tsp. ghee
- Few springs of basil, tarragon, dill, and parsley

Instructions:

1. Pour the herbs and water into the instant pot. Place a trivet into the pot and gently place the salmon onto it.
2. Drizzle the fish with the ghee, pepper, and salt. Cover with slices of the lemon.
3. Lock the lid. Press STEAM to cook for 3 minutes.
4. Julienne your veggies while the salmon cooks.

5. Perform the quick release. Press CANCEL. Remove the rack with the salmon.

6. Discard the herbs. To pot, add veggies. Press SAUTÉ and cook for 1-2 minutes.

7. Serve the salmon with the veggies, along with a teaspoon of the cooking fats if you so choose.

Beef and Broccoli

Calories: 259 Sugar: 2g Carbs: 12g Total Fat: 9g Protein: 28g

Ingredients:

- ¼ tsp. fresh ginger
- 1 tbsp. cooking oil
- 10 to 12-ounce flank steak or sirloin
- 2 minced garlic cloves
- 3 ½ cups broccoli florets
- water

Marinade:

- 1 tsp. cornstarch
- ¼ tsp. dark soy sauce

Jason Michaels

- ½ tsp. sesame oil
- 1 tsp. soy sauce, low-sodium
- 1/8 tsp. pepper

Sauce:

- ¼ tsp. dark soy sauce
- ½ tsp. dry sherry
- 1 tsp. sesame oil, toasted
- 1 ½ tbsp. oyster flavored sauce
- 1 ½ tsp. soy sauce, low-sodium
- 1/3 cup water, cold
- 2 tsp. cornstarch
- 2 tsp. sugar

Instructions:

1. Mix all marinade ingredients together. Add the beef slices and let them sit for at least 10 minutes.
2. Blanch the broccoli.
3. Combine all sauce ingredients together.
4. Warm the oil in either a pan or wok. Add the beef in a single layer to sear. Pour the garlic and continue cooking the meat till cooked through. Pour the sauce in, constantly stirring till it becomes thickened. Add

more water to thin it out if needed. Add the broccoli and stir everything well to coat. Season with the pepper and salt if desired.

5. Sprinkle the sesame seeds and chopped onions if desired.
6. Divide among containers.

Shrimp With Zucchini Noodles

Calories: 119 Sugar: 1g Carbs: 4g Total Fat: 8g Protein: 14g

Ingredients:

- ½ pound shrimp
- 1 tbsp. olive oil
- 4 zucchinis, spiralized

Sauce:

- ¼ cup + 2 tbsps. Thai sweet chili sauce
- ¼ cup + 2 tbsps. light mayo
- ¼ cup + 2 tbsps. plain Greek yogurt
- 1 ½ tsp. sriracha sauce
- 1 ½ tbsp. honey
- 2 tsp. lime juice

Instructions:

1. Cook the shrimp till opaque.
2. Warm up the oil in a pan and add the zucchini till tenderized. Drain and let it rest for 10 minutes.
3. Mix all sauce components together until smooth.
4. Split up the sauce into the containers. Add the zucchini noodles and gently stir to coat well. Add in the shrimp among containers.

Shrimp Taco

Calories: 215 Sugar: 1g Carbs: 3g Total Fat: 15g Protein: 12g

Ingredients:

Spicy Shrimp:

- ¼ tsp. onion powder
- ¼ tsp. salt
- ½ tsp. cumin
- ½ tsp. chili powder
- 1 tbsp. olive oil
- 1 clove garlic, minced

- 20 shrimps

For bowl assembly:

- ½ cup cheddar cheese
- 1 cup black beans
- 1 cup tomatoes
- 1 cup corn
- 1 lime
- 2 tbsps. cilantro

Instructions:

1. Mix all of the shrimp spices together. Add the shrimp, tossing gently to coat. Cover and chill for 10-15 minutes or up to 24 hours.
2. In a skillet, warm the oil and add the shrimp. Cook till cooked thoroughly.
3. To assemble the bowls amongst containers, top with five shrimps, a scoop of tomatoes, beans, corn, and a sprinkle of the cheese and cilantro and a lime wedge.

Refrigerate for up to 14 days.

Jason Michaels

Lemon Roasted Salmon With Sweet Potatoes and Broccolini

Calories: 223 Sugar: 3g Carbs: 5g Total Fat: 19g Protein: 19g

Ingredients:

- 1/8 tsp. red pepper flakes and thyme
- ¼ tsp. garlic powder
- Pepper and salt
- 2 tbsps. lemon juice
- 1 tbsp. butter
- 12 ounces of wild-caught salmon filets
- 4 cups broccoli florets
- 1-3 tbsps. olive oil
- ½ tsp. cumin
- 2 sweet potatoes, cubed

Instructions:

- Ensure the oven is preheated to 425 degrees. On a sheet pan, place the sweet potatoes on one side and the broccoli on the other. Drizzle both with the oil to the pepper, salt, and cumin and toss. Bake the potatoes for 15 minutes and put the broccoli to the side.

- Mix the pepper, salt, thyme, pepper flakes, garlic powder, lemon juice, and butter together. Heat for a few seconds in the microwave for the butter to melt.
- With the foil, line a tray, spray, and place the salmon on it. Drizzle the fish with the lemon sauce.
- Remove the potatoes, put the broccoli and salmon on the tray, and put back in the oven for another 12-15 minutes.
- Divide the veggies and fish among containers.

Dessert Recipes

Cinnamon Apples

Calories: 102 Carbs: 4g Total Fat: 3g Sodium: 24mg Sugar: 32g Protein: 13g

Ingredients:

- ½ cup brown sugar
- 1 tbsp. cinnamon
- 2 tbsps. unsalted butter
- ½ cup sugar
- 1/8 tsp. nutmeg

- 3 tbsps. cornstarch
- 6 Granny Smith apples
- Pinch of salt

Instructions:

1. Peel and thinly slice the apples.
2. Pour all ingredients into your instant pot. Stir well to combine.
3. Press MANUAL to cook for 18 minutes. Perform the natural release.
4. Stir up the mixture well and serve!

Refrigerate for 7 days or freeze for 2 months.

Stuffed Peaches

Calories: 237 Sodium: 173mg Carbs: 8g Sugar: 36g Total Fat: 11g Protein: 15g

Ingredients:

- Pinch of sea salt
- ¼ tsp. almond extract
- ½ tsp. cinnamon

- 2 tbsps. butter
- ¼ cup maple syrup
- ¼ cup cassava flour
- 5 peaches
- ½ cup slivered almonds

Instructions:

1. Cut off about ¼ inch from the top of the peaches. Remove the pits and hollow them all out.
2. Mix together the remaining components till crumbly. Pour the crumble mixture into the peaches.
3. Place a steamer basket into the instant pot. Add 2 cups of the water and place the peaches into the basket.
4. Lock the lid, press MANUAL to cook for 3 minutes. Perform the quick release.
5. Remove the peaches and allow to cool for 10 minutes.

Can be refrigerated for 4 days.

Blackberry Curd

Jason Michaels

Calories: 91 Sugar: 28g Carbs: 2g Total Fat: 0g Sodium: 11mg Protein: 1g

Ingredients:

- 2 tbsps. lemon juice
- 1 cup sugar
- 12 ounces fresh blackberries
- 2 egg yolks
- 2 tbsps. butter

Instructions:

1. Pour the lemon juice, sugar, and blackberries into an instant pot. Lock the lid. Press HIGH PRESSURE to cook for a minute.
2. For 5 minutes, perform the natural pressure release. Then quick release any remaining pressure.
3. Puree the blackberries and remove the seeds as best as you can.
4. Whisk the egg yolks and then add to the hot blackberry puree. Pour it back into the instant pot.
5. Press SAUTÉ and bring to a boil. Stir frequently. Turn off the instant pot and mix in the butter.
6. Pour into the storage container and allow to cool. Chill in the fridge until ready to eat!

Refrigerate for 7 days and freeze for up to 3 months.

'

Cinnamon Pecan Chia Bars

Calories: 175 Sugar: 9g Carbs: 15g Total Fat: 11g Sodium: 143mg Protein: 12g

Ingredients:

- ¼ cup almond butter
- ½ cup pecan pieces
- ¾ tsp. cinnamon
- 2 tbsps. chia seeds
- 12 Medjool dates, pitted

Instructions:

1. With the parchment paper, line a loaf pan. Allow the excess paper to hang over sides for easier removal later on.
2. In a blender, pour in all recipe components. Process till evenly distributed. The mixture should hold its shape.

3. In a loaf pan, pour mixture in. Firmly press into a block that is ½-inch thick. It will more than likely not take up the whole pan.

Chill for 45 minutes till the mixture has set. Slice into the bars.

Chocolate Coconut Bites

Calories: 71 Sugar: 1g Carbs: 21g Total Fat: 16g Sodium: 196mg Protein: 7g

Ingredients:

- ½ cup pecans
- 1 tbsp. cocoa powder
- ½ cup shredded coconut flakes, unsweetened
- 1 tbsp. milk, almond
- 1 tbsp. chia seeds
- 1 tbsp. collagen peptides
- 1 tbsp. liquid coconut oil
- 2 tbsps. hemp seeds
- 8 dates, pitted
- Extra coconut flakes (optional)

Instructions:

1. Blend all recipe components within a food processor till well incorporated.
2. Roll the mixture into 1-inch balls. Roll in additional coconut flakes if you so choose.

Freeze for up to 60 days.

Oatmeal Energy Bites

Calories: 71 Sugar: 1g Carbs: 21g Total Fat: 16g Sodium: 196mg Protein: 7g

Ingredients:

- ½ cup almond butter
- ¼ cup ground flax seed
- 1 cup oats, rolled
- 1/3 cup honey, raw
- ½ cup chocolate chips

Instructions:

1. Mix all recipe components together.
2. Roll out teaspoon-sized balls onto a tray lined with the parchment paper.

3. Freeze the balls for 1 hour.

Freeze for up to 1 month.

Fat Bomb Recipes

Walnut Orange Chocolate Bombs

Calories: 87 Sugar: 1g Carbs: 2g Total Fat: 9g Protein: 2g

Ingredients:

- ¼ cup extra virgin coconut oil
- ½-1 tbsp. orange peel or orange extract
- 1 ¾ cup chopped walnuts
- 1 tsp. cinnamon
- 10-15 drops stevia
- 125 g 85% cocoa dark chocolate

Instructions:

1. Melt the chocolate with your choice of method.
2. Add the cinnamon and coconut oil. Sweeten the mixture with the stevia.
3. Pour in the fresh orange peel and chop the walnuts.

4. In a muffin tin or in the candy cups, spoon in the mixture.

5. Place in the fridge for 1-3 hours until the mixture is solid.

Mini Lemon Tart Bombs

Calories: 101 Protein: 3g Carbs: 1g Total Fat: 11g

Ingredients:

Crust:

- ¾ cup grated dried coconut
- 1 ½ tsp. vanilla extract
- 1 cup almond, cashew or other nut flour
- 2 tbsps. sugar substitute
- 3 tbsps. lemon juice
- 4 ½ tbsps. melted ghee
- Pinch of salt

Filling:

- ¼ tsp. salt
- 1/3 cup lemon juice
- ½ cup softened butter or ghee

Jason Michaels

- 1 tbsp. sugar substitute
- 1/3 cup full-fat almond or coconut milk
- zest of 2 lemons
- 1 tsp. sugar-free vanilla extract
- 2 tsp. lemon extract

Instructions:

1. *For the crust:* Combine entirely crust ingredients in a medium-sized bowl together. Then roll into a log shape with the help of the waxed paper.
2. Proceed to cut into 20-24 slices.
3. Roll each slice into a ball and press gently into the tart pans.
4. Chill until you are ready to fill the crusts.

5. *For the filling:* In a food processor, pour in the butter and beat till fluffy in the texture.
6. Add the salt, zest, extracts, sweetener, lemon juice, and milk, blending until smooth.
7. Taste the mixture periodically and add more lemon juice or sweetener until it meets your taste bud needs.
8. Then pour the filling into your frozen crusts.
9. Top with a sprinkle of the lemon zest.

10. Chill until the tarts are set. Should make about 24 tarts.

Cinnamon Roll Bomb Bars

Calories: 102 Carbs: 2g Total Fat: 15g Protein: 2g

Ingredients:

- ½ cup creamed coconut
- 1/8 tsp. cinnamon

First icing:

- 1 tbsp. butter, almond
- 1 tbsp. coconut oil, extra-virgin

Second icing:

- ½ tsp. cinnamon
- 1 tbsp. coconut oil (extra virgin) or almond butter

Instructions:

1. With the liners, line a mini loaf pan or baking dish.

2. Using your clean hands, combine the cinnamon and coconut cream. Then pat into a dish.

3. In a separate bowl, mix almond butter and coconut oil together. Then spread the mixture over the creamed coconut.

4. Place in the freezer for 5-10 minutes.

5. In yet another bowl, whisk together ingredients of second icing until combined. Drizzle the icing over bars and let it freeze again for 10-20 minutes.

6. Cut into bars and enjoy!

Can be frozen for up to 3 months.

Macadamia Chocolate Fudge Bombs

Calories: 267 Protein: 3g Carbs: 3g Total Fat: 19g

Ingredients:

- ¼ cup heavy cream or coconut oil
- 2 tbsps. sweetener of choice
- 2 ounces cocoa butter
- 2 tbsps. unsweetened cocoa powder
- 4 ounces chopped macadamias

Instructions:

1. In a saucepan, melt the cocoa butter over a simmering pot of water and then add the cocoa powder. Combine.
2. Pour in the sweetener and macadamia nuts and stir well.
3. Then add the cream, mixing well and bringing the mixture back to room temperature.
4. Pour the mixture into the molds or candy cups. Allow time for the bombs to cool and chill to harden.

Peanut Butter Chocolate Bombs

Calories: 211 Protein: 3.5g Carbs: 2g Total Fat: 15g

Ingredients:

- ¼ cup chopped walnuts
- ½ cup butter or coconut oil
- ½ cup natural peanut butter, plain or chunky
- ½ tsp. vanilla extract
- 1 cup sweetener of choice
- 1/3 cup powder, cocoa

- 2 ounces cream cheese, softened
- 1/3 cup vanilla whey powder
- Dash of salt

Instructions:

1. Line a 5 x 7 dish with the parchment paper, ensuring there is an overhang of paper of two sides to aid in the removal later on. Spread the melted butter over the paper as well.
2. In a saucepan on low heat setting, melt the butter and peanut butter together, combining well.
3. In another bowl, beat the cream cheese until it soft and proceed to beat in the peanut butter until smoothened mixture.
4. Add sugar substitute and vanilla.
5. Mix together the salt, protein powder and cocoa powder in a separate bowl, sifting dry ingredients into wet ones until smooth in texture. Stir in nuts.
6. Spread the fudge mixture into the prepared pan, placing in the freezer to harden.
7. Remove and cut into squares. Store in the chilled area before serving.

Savory Mediterranean Fat Bombs

Calories: 164 Protein: 4g Carbs: 2g Total Fat: 17g

Ingredients:

- ¼ cup butter or ghee
- ¼ tsp. salt
- ½ cup full-fat cream cheese
- 2 crushed garlic cloves,
- 2-3 tbsps. freshly chopped herbs
- 4 pieces of drained sun-dried tomatoes
- 4 pitted olives
- 5 tbsps. grated parmesan cheese

Instructions:

1. In a bowl, cut butter into tiny pieces. Then add cream cheese.
2. Let it sit in room temperature for 20-30 minutes until soft.
3. Mash together with the fork until mixed. Add the tomatoes and olives.
4. Add the garlic and herbs, and season to taste with the salt and pepper.
5. Mix well ingredients together.
6. Put in the fridge for 20-30 minutes until solidified.

7. Take out the mixture and form five small balls. Then proceed to the roll balls into the grated parmesan cheese.

8. Eat right away or store in the fridge.

Bacon Guac Bombs

Calories: 156 Protein: 5g Carbs: 1g Total Fat: 15g

Ingredients:

- 4 slices of bacon
- ¼ tsp. salt
- 1 tbsp. lime fresh lime juice
- ½ small diced onion
- 1 chopped chili pepper
- 2 cloves crushed garlic
- ¼ cup butter or ghee
- ½ large avocado
- 1-2 tbsps. freshly chopped cilantro
- 1/8 tsp. cayenne pepper

Instructions:

1. Ensure the oven is preheated to 375 degrees.

2. Using the parchment paper, line a baking tray and proceed to lay out the bacon slices, ensuring none overlap.

3. Cook the bacon for 10-15 minutes or until golden brown. Remove and let it cool.

4. In a bowl, mash together the remaining ingredients together until combined. Then add diced onion.

5. Add the bacon grease and combine. Cover the mixture with the foil and put into the fridge for 20-30 minutes.

6. Crumble the bacon to use as breading.

7. Roll the avocado mixture into about six balls and roll into bacon pieces.

Salmon Bombs

Calories: 147 Protein: 3g Carbs: 0.5g Total Fat: 16g

Ingredients:

- ½ cup cream cheese, full-fat
- 1 tbsp. lemon juice, fresh
- ½ package smoked salmon or smoked mackerel
- 1/3 cup butter
- 1-2 tbsps. chopped fresh or dried dill

Instructions:

1. In a food processor, pour in salmon, butter, and cream cheese, adding the lemon juice and dill while pulsing.
2. With the parchment paper, line a tray and place the salmon mixture in 2.5 tablespoon sizes on the tray.
3. Top with the dill and put in the fridge to chill for 1-2 hours until firm.

Jalapeno and Cheese Bombs

Calories: 142 Protein: 4g Carbs: 1g Total Fat: 15g

Ingredients:

- ¼ cup grated cheddar cheese
- ¼ cup unsalted butter
- 2 g halved, seeded, & chopped jalapeño peppers
- 3.5 ounces of full-fat cream cheese
- 4 slices of bacon

Instructions:

1. Ensure your oven is preheated to 325 degrees.

2. With the parchment paper, line a baking sheet, ensuring there is extra hanging over the edge to aid in removing later.

3. Mash together the cream cheese and butter in a bowl and then put in the food processor, mix until smooth in texture.

4. Lay out the bacon slices on the parchment paper, leaving a space between them. Cook for 25-30 minutes until the slices are crispy. Remove and set aside to allow to cool.

5. Add together the cheese and jalapeños to the cream cheese and butter mixture. Chill for half an hour to 1 hour until set.

6. Split up the mixture into six fat bombs and place them on the parchment paper. If serving right away, roll in the crumbled bacon. If later, chill the mixture before coating in the bacon.

Pizza Bombs

Calories: 112 Protein: 5g Carbs: 2g Total Fat: 10.5g

Ingredients:

- 14 slices of pepperoni
- 2 tbsps. freshly chopped basil

- 2 tbsps. sun-dried tomato pesto
- 4 ounces of cream cheese
- 8 pitted black olives

Instructions:

1. Chop up the olives and pepperoni.
2. In a bowl, mix all together the cream cheese, tomato pesto, and basil and add the pepperoni and olives, mixing well to combine.
3. Form the mixture into balls and then top with the pepperoni, basil, and olive.

Rice Alternatives

One of the toughest challenges when doing keto is finding substitutes for plain old white rice. Here's 10 easy ones.

Cauliflower Rice
Just mince up cauliflower to a rice-like consistency in a food processor and you're good to go. One serving even contains a day's worth of Vitamin C

Broccoli Rice
Same as above - also looks great for photos!

Green Bean Fries

Sauteed green beans with some garlic and olive oil go well with so many different meals.

Zucchini Noodles

A great way to add some more bulk to meals, ideal if you naturally need to eat a higher volume of food to stay full. Use a spiralizer to make these.

Butternut Squash Noodles

Same as above

...and the one food which isn't keto friendly - but everyone thinks is...

Quinoa!

Whether it's red, black or white quinoa, all of these have more than 30g of net carbs per serving, and as such, will usually break your state of ketosis. Avoid quinoa if you're doing keto.

Jason Michaels

Emergency Keto Meals at Popular Fast Food Chains

As much as we like to plan, it's not possible to stay consistent 100% of the time. Life gets in the way. Fortunately, most fast food chains now have keto friendly meals. Here's a few options at the big chains.

Subway

Skip the bread (duh) and opt for a salad instead. The tuna salad with cheese, black olives, green peppers, lettuce, spinach and pickles has just 330 calories and 7G net carbs. Don't bother with dressings or sauces outside of olive oil, salt and pepper - and you're good to go

Chipotle

A salad bowl with meat, tomato based salsa (no corn), sour cream and cheese is both delicious and keto-approved.

McDonald's

Pro-tip, you can order the sandwiches without bread! Some restaurants might give you a strange look. Worst case scenario you order normally and toss out the bun. The

McDouble, McChicken and Grilled Chicken Sandwich are all keto friendly. As are the sausage and egg mcmuffins

Burger King

Same applies here, a Whopper or Double Cheeseburger without bread or ketchup is keto friendly.

Taco Bell

This one is a little more complicated - order a side of lettuce, side of beef, side of chicken, and side or two of guacamole, then combine for a quick and cheap meal.

KFC

Protein heaven over at the colonel. Grilled chicken thighs are 17g protein with 0 carbs per piece. Breasts are 38g with no carbs. You can also get a side of green beans.

Carl's Jr.

One of the few places which actually has Lettuce-wrapped as an option. The thick burger is just 9G of carbs when you opt for this keto-friendly choice.

Jason Michaels

Jimmy John's

Any of their sandwiches can be made as Unwiches (order a slim one if you want a save a few bucks) which means no bread.

Five Guys

Same as Carl's Jr. Just order the lettuce wrap options and you're good to go.

In-n-Out

Order your burger "protein style" - a hamburger, cheeseburger or double double comes it at 11G of net carbs with this method.

Chapter 5: Methods to Properly Store Food

Congratulations! So far you know the ins and outs of the ketogenic diet, meal prep mistakes to avoid, and a nice array of keto meal prep recipes to get you started! Now, it's time to discover the proper way to store your deliciously prepped meals so that you can enjoy them as if they were fresh off the press!

Pantry Tips

There are many other items besides fruits, veggies, and canned goods that can reside happily in a pantry. These tips pertain to the foods in storage that don't need to be frozen or refrigerated:

- To lengthen the time of prepper foods, store them in the plastic or glass meal prep containers

- Most canned foods that are low in acid, such as vegetables, crab meat, and tuna can last up to 2 to 5 years. Ensure you check the date.

- Canned foods that are high in acid, like the tomato-based items, pineapple, and grapefruit have a shelf life of 12 to 18 months.

- Conditions of storage areas should be cool, dark, and dry with temperatures that range from 50 to 70 degrees. Warm climate makes the food deteriorate faster, so keep the items away from the hot pipes, dishwasher, and oven.

Fridge Tips

- Stay alert for spoiled food. If anything looks or smells off, it should be thrown out. Yes, mold can happen in the fridge too.

- Keep the prepped meals covered and in the plastic or glass containers, wrapped in the foil or plastic wrap.

- Pay attention to the expiration dates.

- Be vigilant of the 2-hour rule of refrigeration, meaning not leaving items that require to be chilled out for more than 2 hours, such as dairy, seafood, eggs, meat, chicken, etc.

- Set the temperature in your fridge to 40 degrees or lower.

Freezer Tips

I want to nicely remind you that freezing meals does not kill bacteria, but it can stop it from growing. Most frozen foods can last for a long time, but the color, flavor, and tenderness of the frozen items can be affected the longer they are frozen.

- Thaw food in your fridge before prepping

- Don't fear the freezer burn; it's a quality of food issue, not a food safety problem

- Label all packages you freeze with the date, what food is in it, and any other identifying information that will help your meal prep efforts, such as what it weighs or how many servings are in the container

- Ensure that you properly wrap the food you wish to freeze, utilize the airtight storage containers, and use the bags, plastic wrap, and foil that is freezer-grade

- Set the temperature of your freezer to 0 degrees or below

Freezer vs. Fridge

Not all edibles are freezer friendly:

- Fruits high in water content
- Lettuce
- Uncooked batters
- Eggs
- Cooked pasta
- Soft cheeses
- Cultured dairy

Freeze your meals if you don't plan to consume them in 3 to 4 days after you prepare them. Remember that the prepping frozen meals take a bit more preparation time than refrigerated meals.

- Thaw out meals for a few hours or overnight before heating and consuming

- Frozen meals last substantially longer than refrigerated meals, some being able to be frozen up to 1 year

Refrigerated meals are capable of being tasty, fresh, and convenient for a few days. After prepping, you just have to nuke the meals in the microwave. After several days of living in the fridge, however, meals can lose their freshness, taste, and moisture. This is because dry air circulating takes the moisture out of the food.

Refrigerate the meals you plan to eat in 3 to 4 days.

Chapter 6: Meal Prep Kitchen Essentials

Setting the time aside each week to prep meals for the entire week is a great way to eliminate the cravings for unhealthy eats and keep you on the right track to achieving your health and fitness goals.

Many people avoid the task of meal planning and prepping simply because they think of it as another chore; this is because they are using the wrong kitchen tools to get this big job done. This chapter will share the essential tools you need to simplify the process of meal prepping and make it more manageable.

High-quality knives

One of the most crucial tools to meal prep is having a decent set of knives that allow you to slice, dice, chop, and chiffonade like a master chef! If you have dull knives in your kitchen drawers, you are *asking* for prepping disaster. Sharp knives will save you time and make meal prep a lot easier on your hands. I recommend <u>stainless steel knives</u> for longevity!

Measuring spoons and cups

If you are meal prepping around macro measurements, it's very crucial to ensure you are measuring correctly. Measuring cups can help you measure dry ingredients like nuts and seeds while measuring spoons will help measure spices.

Food scale

Even though the majority of people can easily get away with measuring with cups and spoons, there are some people that need to ensure accuracy with a food scale. These are also helpful to measure proteins.

Good kitchen utensils

Having good quality kitchen utensils is obviously essential for breezing through meal prep! When you have well-rounded utensils, you can better prepare a variety of meals with ease.

Cutting boards

Almost all meal prep recipes involve dicing, cutting, or chopping, so you need one of these at arm's length always.

Mixing bowls

Jason Michaels

Good mixing bowls are used to mix batters, marinate proteins, and much more.

Colander

Good for draining veggies and aiming for clean-tasting produce. You want crispy, rainbow-like vegetables, right?

Grater

Meal preppers love graters! It allows them to add lots of flavors to any recipe with a few simple swipes. Zest a lemon, shave some chocolate, grate a bit of nutmeg, etc.

Baking dishes

- Round cake pans
- 13 x 9 baking sheet
- 8 x 8 and 9 x 5 loaf pans
- Muffin pans
- Etc.

Non-stick skillet

Skillets are highly versatile, and you can cook just about anything in them with a little bit of fat.

Cast iron skillet

An amazing gadget for the keto diet, this skillet is capable of adding flavor and iron to your meals.

Sauté pans

Saucepan with lid

Sheet pans

Roasting pan

Cook an amazing evening meal that makes a ton of leftovers! You can even make extremely large batches of items such as granola.

Cooling rack

Spiralizer

Obviously regular pasta is not keto friendly, but a better, healthier alternative can be created with the help of spiralizing vegetables like zucchini. Yum!

Food Processor

Jason Michaels

Don't want to chop your veggies? Stick them in a food processor! Great for making pesto, hummus, dips, shredding chicken, etc.

Crockpot

Crock pots are a meal prepper's *dream* appliance; if you want to further your meal prep skills, you can save even *more* time with these babies and can make a large variety of meals and desserts.

High-speed blender

No matter if you are making the nut butter, sauces, soups, or smoothies, a good blender is a must and can help you blend in seconds!

Meal prep containers

Quality meal prep containers are an essential staple to the meal planning world. You want ones that are durable and that you can use consistently for a long period of time. Opt for containers with lockable lids rather than the standard lids which can fall off because of condensation.

www.ingramcontent.com/pod-product-compliance
Lightning Source LLC
Chambersburg PA
CBHW060315030426
42336CB00011B/1053